KIDNEY DISEASE DIET FOOD LIST FOR SENIORS ON STAGE 4

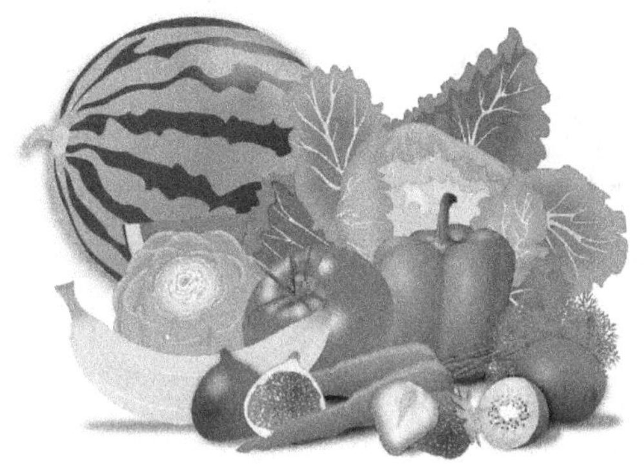

A Simple and Easy Low Phosphorus, Low Potassium and Low Sodium foods to Support CKD Management

EDITH GONZALES

TABLE OF CONTENTS

How to Use This Book

This book is designed to be a comprehensive guide for seniors with stage 4 chronic kidney disease (CKD), providing valuable information on dietary management, meal planning, and food selection to help manage your condition. Here's how you can make the most out of this resource:

1. Understand Your Dietary Needs
Before diving into the food lists and recipes, it's essential to understand the dietary requirements specific to stage 4 CKD. This includes managing the intake of key nutrients such as sodium, potassium, phosphorus, and protein, which can impact kidney function and overall health. Familiarize yourself with the dietary guidelines provided in the introduction to grasp why certain foods are recommended and others are to be avoided.

2. Navigate the Food Lists
The book is organized into sections that categorize foods based on their nutrient content and suitability for a stage 4 CKD diet. Each list provides a selection of foods that are low in sodium, potassium, phosphorus, or protein, making it easier to plan your meals.

➤ Vegetables and Fruits: Learn which low-potassium and low-phosphorus fruits and vegetables are safe to include in your diet, and understand the serving sizes to maintain nutrient balance.

➤ Grains and Proteins: Discover grains and protein sources that are kidney-friendly, focusing on those that are low in phosphorus and potassium. The lists help you choose the right carbohydrates and protein sources to meet your nutritional needs without overloading your kidneys.

➤ Dairy Alternatives and Snacks: Explore options for dairy alternatives and snacks that won't contribute to phosphorus or sodium overload, providing healthy and satisfying options throughout the day.

➤ Herbs and Spices: Find out how to flavor your meals without adding extra sodium, and see which herbs and spices are safe to use in a CKD diet.

3. Use the Recipes for Meal Planning
In addition to food lists, the book includes recipes specifically crafted for seniors with stage 4 CKD. These recipes provide detailed nutritional information, including the

amounts of phosphorus, sodium, and potassium per serving. This allows you to track your nutrient intake accurately and helps you create balanced meals that fit your dietary restrictions.

> ➤ Breakfast, Lunch, and Dinner Recipes: Each meal category offers a variety of recipes to ensure you have options for every meal of the day. These recipes are designed to be simple to prepare, making meal planning easier.

> ➤ Snacks and Sides: Use these recipes to add variety and ensure you have healthy options between meals without overloading on restricted nutrients.

> ➤ Beverages and Desserts: Enjoy beverages and treats that are kidney-friendly, allowing you to indulge without compromising your diet.

4. Incorporate Meal Planning Tips
Meal planning is a crucial aspect of managing stage 4 CKD. The book offers tips on how to plan your meals effectively, taking into account your daily nutrient limits. Use these tips to organize your grocery shopping, prepare meals in advance, and ensure you're adhering to your dietary plan consistently.

5. Adjust and Monitor
Your dietary needs may change over time, especially as CKD progresses. It's important to regularly monitor your health and adjust your diet accordingly. This book can serve as a reference to revisit and modify your food choices as needed.

> Tracking Intake: Utilize the detailed nutritional information provided to keep track of your daily intake of sodium, potassium, phosphorus, and protein. This can help you stay within the recommended limits and avoid complications.

> Consultation with Healthcare Providers: Always discuss any dietary changes with your healthcare provider or dietitian. Use this book as a tool to support those discussions, ensuring that your diet is tailored to your current health status.

6. Stay Informed and Empowered
This book is not just a list of foods but a resource to empower you to make informed dietary decisions. Understanding the reasons behind food choices and being proactive in your meal planning can significantly impact your health and well-being.

Use this book as an ongoing resource, adapting your diet as needed and staying informed about the best practices for managing stage 4 CKD.

Overview of Stage 4 Chronic Kidney Disease (CKD)

Stage 4 Chronic Kidney Disease (CKD) represents a critical stage where kidney function is significantly compromised, with a glomerular filtration rate (GFR) between 15 and 29 mL/min. At this stage, the kidneys are no longer able to effectively filter waste and excess fluids from the blood, which can lead to the accumulation of toxins and the need for careful dietary management. For seniors, who may have additional health concerns, adhering to a kidney-friendly diet is essential to managing symptoms, slowing disease progression, and maintaining overall well-being.

Importance of a Kidney Disease Diet

A kidney disease diet is tailored to minimize the intake of certain nutrients that the kidneys can no longer effectively regulate, such as sodium, potassium, phosphorus, and protein. The diet also ensures adequate caloric intake to prevent malnutrition while reducing the risk of complications like hyperkalemia (high potassium levels), hyperphosphatemia (high phosphorus levels), and hypertension (high blood pressure). For seniors, a kidney-friendly diet can improve quality of life, support energy levels, and help manage other chronic conditions that often accompany aging.

Key Nutritional Considerations

1. Sodium:

Sodium is commonly found in salt and processed foods. Excessive sodium intake can lead to fluid retention, swelling, and increased blood pressure, all of which put additional strain on the kidneys. Seniors with stage 4 CKD should aim to limit sodium intake to 1,500 to 2,000 mg per day.

2. Potassium:

Potassium is vital for muscle function and heart health, but in stage 4 CKD, the kidneys struggle to balance potassium levels, which can lead to dangerous heart rhythms. Limiting potassium intake is crucial, with typical recommendations ranging from 2,000 to 3,000 mg per day, depending on individual blood levels.

3. Phosphorus:

Phosphorus, found in many foods, especially dairy, nuts, and whole grains, can accumulate in the blood when kidney function is impaired. High phosphorus levels can lead to bone and cardiovascular issues. Seniors should aim to limit phosphorus intake to around 800 to 1,000 mg per day.

4. Protein:

While protein is essential for body repair and maintenance, excessive protein intake can increase the burden on the kidneys. In stage 4 CKD, protein intake is typically limited to about 0.6 to 0.8 grams per kilogram of body weight per day, depending on individual needs.

5. Fluid Intake:

Fluid intake must be carefully monitored, especially if there is reduced urine output. Seniors should follow the guidelines provided by their healthcare provider, which may involve restricting fluids to prevent fluid overload.

Creating a Balanced Diet:

The key to managing stage 4 CKD through diet is careful planning and selecting foods that are low in sodium, potassium, and phosphorus, while providing adequate nutrition. A kidney-friendly diet for seniors should include a variety of foods from all food groups in appropriate portions:

> Fruits and Vegetables: Focus on low-potassium options such as apples, berries, cauliflower, and green beans. These provide essential vitamins and fiber while keeping potassium levels in check.

> Grains and Starches: Opt for white rice, pasta, and bread over whole grains to reduce phosphorus intake. These foods can provide energy without overloading the kidneys.

> Proteins: Choose high-quality protein sources in limited quantities, such as eggs, lean poultry, and fish. Plant-based proteins like tofu and low-potassium beans can also be included in moderation.

> Dairy Alternatives: Use low-phosphorus dairy alternatives like rice milk or almond milk instead of regular milk. These provide essential nutrients without the high phosphorus content.

> Fats and Oils: Healthy fats like olive oil, flaxseed oil, and small amounts of butter or margarine can be used to add flavor and calories.

> Herbs and Spices: Instead of salt, use herbs and spices like garlic, onion powder, basil, and rosemary to enhance the flavor of meals without increasing sodium intake.

Meal Planning and Portion Control:

For seniors with stage 4 CKD, portion control is crucial to managing nutrient intake. Meals should be balanced and portioned according to individual needs, with an emphasis on variety to ensure all essential nutrients are included. It is also important to read food labels and be aware of hidden sources of sodium, potassium, and phosphorus in processed foods.

The Role of Medical Endorsement and Monitoring:

A kidney disease diet should always be tailored and supervised by a healthcare provider or a registered dietitian who specializes in renal nutrition. Regular monitoring of blood levels and overall health is essential to adjust dietary intake as needed. For seniors, regular check-ups and blood tests are critical to ensure that the diet is effectively managing the disease and maintaining health.

Food to limits or avoid for Seniors with stage 4 CkD

For seniors with stage 4 Chronic Kidney Disease (CKD), the kidneys are significantly impaired, leading to an inability to effectively filter waste products and balance electrolytes. As a result, certain foods can exacerbate symptoms and contribute to complications. It's crucial to limit or avoid specific foods to manage the disease and prevent further kidney damage.

1. High-Potassium Foods
Why Limit: The kidneys in stage 4 CKD struggle to remove excess potassium from the blood, leading to hyperkalemia, a condition that can cause muscle weakness, irregular heartbeats, and potentially life-threatening heart conditions.

Foods to Avoid:
1. Fruits: Bananas, oranges, cantaloupe, honeydew, avocado, kiwi, and dried fruits (raisins, prunes).
2. Vegetables: Potatoes (including sweet potatoes), tomatoes, spinach, broccoli, and mushrooms.
3. Other: Coconut water, tomato-based sauces, and high-potassium salt substitutes.
4. Alternative Choices: Opt for low-potassium fruits like apples, berries, grapes, and low-potassium vegetables like cauliflower, bell peppers, and zucchini.

2. High-Phosphorus Foods

Why Limit: Phosphorus levels can rise when kidney function declines, leading to weakened bones and the risk of cardiovascular disease due to calcium-phosphorus deposits in the body.

Foods to Avoid:
1. Dairy Products: Milk, cheese, yogurt, ice cream, and custards.
2. Processed Foods: Colas, packaged snacks, fast food, and foods with added phosphates (check labels for "phosphoric acid" or "phosphate").

3. Protein Sources: Organ meats, sardines, nuts, seeds, and whole grains like brown rice and whole wheat bread.
4. Alternative Choices: Use dairy alternatives like rice milk or almond milk, and choose low-phosphorus snacks like unsalted popcorn or rice cakes.

3. High-Sodium Foods

Why Limit: Sodium can cause fluid retention, increasing blood pressure and worsening swelling and heart strain, all of which can further impair kidney function.

Foods to Avoid:
1. Processed Meats: Bacon, ham, sausages, hot dogs, and deli meats.
2. Canned and Packaged Foods: Soups, vegetables, and frozen dinners that are high in sodium.
3. Snack Foods: Potato chips, pretzels, salted nuts, and crackers.
4. Condiments: Soy sauce, pickles, olives, and salad dressings.
5. Alternative Choices: Use fresh or frozen vegetables without added salt, and flavor food with herbs and spices instead of salt. Choose low-sodium versions of processed foods when available.

4. High-Protein Foods

Why Limit: While protein is essential, excessive intake can produce more waste products that the kidneys need to filter, increasing their workload.

Foods to Avoid:

1. Red Meat: Beef, lamb, and pork.
2. Full-Fat Dairy: Cheese, whole milk, and cream.
3. Protein Supplements: Protein powders and shakes that contain high levels of protein.
4. Alternative Choices: Include smaller portions of high-quality protein like eggs, poultry, or fish, and consider plant-based proteins in moderation.

5. Processed and Fast Foods

Why Limit: These foods are often high in sodium, phosphorus, and unhealthy fats, which can lead to fluid retention, increased blood pressure, and further kidney damage.

Foods to Avoid:

1. Fast Food: Burgers, fries, pizza, and fried chicken.
2. Packaged Snacks: Chips, cookies, and pastries.
3. Convenience Meals: Frozen dinners, instant noodles, and packaged mixes.

4. Alternative Choices: Prepare homemade meals using fresh ingredients, and choose whole, unprocessed foods whenever possible.

6. Sugary Foods and Beverages

Why Limit: Excessive sugar intake can lead to weight gain and increased blood sugar levels, which can worsen kidney function and exacerbate conditions like diabetes.

Foods to Avoid:
1. Sugary Drinks: Sodas, sweetened fruit juices, energy drinks, and sugary coffee drinks.
2. Desserts: Cakes, pies, candy, and pastries.
3. Alternative Choices: Opt for water, unsweetened herbal teas, and fruits with low sugar content like berries or apples.

7. Alcohol

Why Limit: Alcohol can dehydrate the body, affect blood pressure, and worsen kidney function, making it especially risky for those with stage 4 CKD.

Beverages to Avoid:
1. Beer: High in phosphorus and can increase fluid load.
2. Wine and Spirits: Can interact with medications and exacerbate kidney strain.
3. Alternative Choices: If alcohol is consumed, it should be in very limited quantities and approved by a healthcare provider.

8. High-Oxalate Foods

Why Limit: High levels of oxalates can lead to the formation of kidney stones, which can be particularly dangerous for those with impaired kidney function.

Foods to Avoid:
1. Leafy Greens: Spinach, rhubarb, and beet greens.
2. Nuts: Almonds, cashews, and peanuts.
3. Other: Chocolate, beets, and sweet potatoes.
4. Alternative Choices: Opt for lower-oxalate vegetables like cabbage, lettuce, and cauliflower.

9. Dark-Colored Colas and Soda
Why Limit: Dark colas contain phosphorus additives, which can contribute to high phosphorus levels and bone health issues in CKD patients.

Beverages to Avoid: All dark colas and sodas with phosphoric acid.
Alternative Choices: Choose clear sodas without phosphorus additives, or better yet, water flavored with lemon or cucumber.

10. Artificial Sweeteners and Preservatives
Why Limit: Some artificial sweeteners and preservatives can strain the kidneys and may contribute to long-term health issues.

Foods to Avoid: Foods and drinks with artificial sweeteners like aspartame, saccharin, and foods high in preservatives.
Alternative Choices: Use natural sweeteners like stevia in moderation and consume fresh, whole foods.

Meal planning Tips for Seniors with Stage 4 CKD

Meal planning for seniors with Stage 4 Chronic Kidney Disease (CKD) is a crucial component of managing the condition and slowing its progression. At this stage, the kidneys are severely impaired, and dietary adjustments are necessary to minimize the buildup of waste products and maintain overall health. Proper meal planning helps in balancing nutrients, avoiding harmful foods, and ensuring that seniors receive adequate calories and nutrition.

1. Understand Nutritional Restrictions
   - Sodium: Limit sodium intake to 1,500-2,000 mg per day to prevent fluid retention and high blood pressure. Avoid adding salt to meals and choose low-sodium versions of foods.

   - Potassium: Keep potassium intake within recommended levels (usually 2,000-3,000 mg/day) by selecting low-potassium fruits and vegetables. Monitor blood levels regularly.

➢ Phosphorus: Limit phosphorus intake to 800-1,000 mg per day to prevent bone and cardiovascular complications. Avoid high-phosphorus foods like dairy products, nuts, and processed foods with added phosphates.

➢ Protein: Moderate protein intake (0.6-0.8 grams per kilogram of body weight) to reduce kidney workload while still supporting muscle maintenance and other bodily functions.

2. Work with a Dietitian
➢ Personalized Plan: A registered dietitian specializing in renal nutrition can help tailor a meal plan that meets the specific needs of seniors with CKD. This personalized approach ensures that nutritional requirements are met while adhering to dietary restrictions.

➢ Regular Adjustments: As kidney function changes, dietary needs may also change. Regular check-ins with a dietitian help in adjusting the meal plan as necessary.

3. Plan Balanced Meals

➢ Variety of Foods: Include a variety of low-sodium, low-potassium, and low-phosphorus foods to ensure a balanced intake of vitamins and minerals. This variety also prevents meal fatigue.

➢ Portion Control: Carefully monitor portion sizes, especially for foods that are higher in potassium, phosphorus, or sodium, to stay within daily limits.

➢ Balanced Plate: Aim for a balanced plate with a moderate amount of protein, a good portion of low-potassium vegetables, a small serving of grains, and a healthy fat source.

4. Focus on Whole Foods

➢ Fresh Ingredients: Use fresh or frozen vegetables and fruits instead of canned or processed ones, which often contain added sodium and preservatives.

➢ Whole Grains and Alternatives: Opt for refined grains like white rice and pasta over whole grains to reduce phosphorus intake. These can still be part of a healthy meal when paired with the right foods.

➢ Minimize Processed Foods: Processed foods often contain hidden sodium, phosphorus, and potassium. Focus on whole, unprocessed foods to maintain control over nutrient intake.

5. Be Cautious with Fluids

➢ Fluid Intake: Seniors with CKD may need to limit fluid intake to prevent fluid overload, especially if urine output is reduced. Include foods with high water content like soups and gelatin in moderation, and monitor total fluid intake throughout the day.

➢ Fluid Planning: If fluid restrictions are in place, divide the allowed fluid intake across the day, and avoid drinking too much at one time.

6. Use Flavor Enhancers Wisely

➢ Herbs and Spices: Use herbs, spices, lemon juice, vinegar, and garlic to flavor foods without adding salt. Avoid seasoning mixes that may contain hidden sodium or potassium.

➢ Low-Sodium Options: Opt for low-sodium or sodium-free condiments, and experiment with salt-free spice blends to enhance the flavor of meals.

7. Plan Ahead for Convenience

➢ Meal Prep: Prepare meals and snacks in advance to make it easier to adhere to dietary restrictions. Batch cooking and portioning meals can save time and ensure that ready-to-eat meals are kidney-friendly.

➢ Label Reading: When buying packaged foods, carefully read labels for sodium, potassium, and phosphorus content. Familiarize yourself with terms like "phosphate" on ingredient lists to avoid hidden phosphorus.

8. Include Healthy Snacks

➢ Low-Potassium Snacks: Choose snacks that are low in potassium and phosphorus, such as unsalted popcorn, rice cakes, or apple slices. These can help maintain energy levels between meals without exceeding nutrient limits.

➢ Controlled Portions: Keep snacks portion-controlled to avoid unintentional overconsumption of restricted nutrients.

9. Consider Nutritional Supplements

➢ Renal Vitamins: Some seniors with CKD may require specific vitamins or supplements to meet their nutritional needs, especially if dietary intake is limited. Renal-specific vitamins are often recommended to avoid excessive potassium and phosphorus.

➤ Protein Supplements: If protein intake is low, protein supplements specifically designed for CKD patients may be helpful. Always consult with a healthcare provider before starting any supplements.

10. Stay Hydrated with Care

➤ Fluid Sources: In addition to drinking water, consider foods with high water content like cucumbers, lettuce, and gelatin as part of the fluid allowance.

➤ Monitor Symptoms: Watch for signs of fluid overload, such as swelling or shortness of breath, and adjust fluid intake accordingly under the guidance of a healthcare provider.

11. Incorporate Small, Frequent Meals

➤ Meal Frequency: Eating smaller, more frequent meals can help manage blood sugar levels, energy levels, and nutrient intake. This approach also prevents overeating at any one meal, which can help control potassium and phosphorus intake.

> Digestive Comfort: Smaller meals can be easier to digest and may prevent discomfort, which is important for seniors with multiple health concerns.

12. Stay Informed and Flexible
> Education: Keep informed about which foods are safe and which to avoid as new research or dietary recommendations emerge. Understanding the reasons behind dietary restrictions can help make more informed food choices.

> Flexibility: Be prepared to adapt meal plans as kidney function changes or as other health conditions arise.

Dietary Guidelines for Seniors with stage 4 CKD

Managing diet is crucial for seniors with stage 4 Chronic Kidney Disease (CKD). At this stage, the kidneys are significantly impaired, meaning they can no longer effectively remove waste products and maintain the body's balance of fluids, electrolytes, and nutrients. Careful dietary planning can help control the progression of CKD, reduce symptoms, and improve the quality of life.

1. Protein Intake
Guideline: Protein intake should be carefully managed to reduce the workload on the kidneys while ensuring enough protein to prevent muscle wasting.

Recommendation:
> Amount: Typically, 0.6 to 0.8 grams of protein per kilogram of body weight per day is recommended for those with stage 4 CKD. This should be adjusted based on individual needs and medical advice.

> Sources: Choose high-quality protein sources such as eggs, fish, chicken, and

small portions of lean meat. Consider including plant-based proteins like tofu and beans in moderation, as they are lower in phosphorus and potassium.

➢ Caution: Avoid high-protein diets and protein supplements unless prescribed by a healthcare provider.

2. Sodium Restriction

Guideline: Sodium intake should be limited to prevent fluid retention, high blood pressure, and heart strain, which are common concerns in CKD.

Recommendation:
➢ Amount: Limit sodium to 1,500 to 2,000 mg per day.

➢ Sources: Focus on fresh, unprocessed foods, and avoid adding salt during cooking or at the table. Be cautious with processed foods, canned goods, pickles, and condiments like soy sauce and salad dressings.

➢ Caution: Always read labels for sodium content, and choose low-sodium or sodium-free options when possible.

3. Potassium Management

Guideline: Managing potassium intake is crucial as the kidneys' ability to excrete potassium diminishes, leading to dangerous levels in the blood.

Recommendation:

> Amount: Potassium intake should typically be limited to 2,000 to 3,000 mg per day, but this should be individualized based on lab results.

> Sources: Opt for low-potassium fruits (like apples, berries, and grapes) and vegetables (such as bell peppers, cabbage, and cauliflower). Avoid high-potassium foods like bananas, oranges, potatoes, tomatoes, and spinach.

> Caution: Be cautious with potassium-rich salt substitutes, and avoid high-potassium foods unless recommended by a dietitian.

4. Phosphorus Control

Guideline: Limit phosphorus intake to prevent bone weakening and cardiovascular issues, as phosphorus can accumulate in the blood when kidney function is reduced.

Recommendation:
> ➢ Amount: Phosphorus intake should be restricted to 800 to 1,000 mg per day.

> ➢ Sources: Avoid foods high in phosphorus, such as dairy products, nuts, seeds, whole grains, and cola beverages. Instead, choose refined grains like white rice and pasta, and low-phosphorus dairy alternatives like rice milk.

> ➢ Caution: Watch out for hidden phosphorus in processed foods and avoid those with ingredients like "phosphate" or "phosphoric acid" listed on the label.

5. Fluid Management

Guideline: Fluid intake may need to be controlled to prevent fluid overload, particularly if urine output is significantly reduced.

Recommendation:
> ➢ Amount: Fluid needs vary based on the individual's condition, but intake may be limited to around 1,000 to 1,500 ml per day if fluid retention is an issue.

➤ Sources: Include the fluid content of foods like soups and gelatin in the daily fluid allowance. Drink water, but avoid high-potassium beverages like orange juice and coconut water.

➤ Caution: Monitor weight daily and report sudden gains, which may indicate fluid overload.

6. Calcium and Vitamin D Intake
Guideline: Calcium and Vitamin D are important for bone health, but their intake should be carefully monitored to avoid complications.

Recommendation:
➤ Sources: Include low-phosphorus calcium sources like fortified rice or almond milk and calcium supplements if prescribed. Ensure adequate vitamin D intake, either through diet or supplements, as recommended by a healthcare provider.

➤ Caution: Avoid excessive calcium supplementation, which can lead to calcification of blood vessels and soft tissues.

7. Carbohydrate and Fat Management
Guideline: Carbohydrates and fats should provide the majority of calories to prevent muscle breakdown, but they should come from healthy sources.

Recommendation:
- ➤ Carbohydrates: Focus on complex carbohydrates like white rice, pasta, and refined grains that are lower in phosphorus. Avoid sugary foods and beverages to prevent weight gain and blood sugar spikes.

- ➤ Fats: Choose healthy fats such as olive oil, avocado, and omega-3 rich fish like salmon, but in moderation.

- ➤ Caution: Limit saturated fats and avoid trans fats to maintain heart health, which is especially important in CKD.

8. Vitamins and Minerals
Guideline: Certain vitamins and minerals may need to be supplemented due to dietary restrictions, but others, like fat-soluble vitamins, should be limited.

Recommendation:
- ➤ Sources: A renal-specific multivitamin may be recommended to ensure

adequate intake of B vitamins, vitamin C, and other essential nutrients without excess potassium or phosphorus.

➢ Caution: Avoid over-the-counter multivitamins that are not specifically formulated for kidney disease, as they may contain high levels of potassium or phosphorus.

9. Meal Timing and Portion Control

Guideline: Eating smaller, more frequent meals can help manage blood sugar levels, control hunger, and prevent overeating, which is important for overall health.

Recommendation:

➢ Meal Frequency: Aim for 5-6 small meals throughout the day instead of 3 large ones to help balance nutrient intake and digestion.

➢ Portion Sizes: Carefully control portions of high-potassium, high-phosphorus, and high-protein foods to stay within daily limits.

10. Limit Processed and Convenience Foods
Guideline: Processed and convenience foods often contain hidden sodium, phosphorus, and unhealthy fats, making them unsuitable for a CKD diet.

Recommendation:
- ➢ Foods to Avoid: Fast food, canned soups, frozen dinners, and packaged snacks. Instead, prepare meals using fresh ingredients to have better control over nutrient content.

- ➢ Healthy Alternatives: When choosing processed foods, opt for those labeled as low-sodium, low-potassium, and phosphorus-free.

11. Monitor and Adjust Diet Regularly
Guideline: Regularly monitor blood work and symptoms to adjust the diet as needed in response to changes in kidney function or overall health.

Recommendation:
- ➢ Collaborate with Healthcare Providers: Regularly consult with a dietitian and nephrologist to tailor the diet to current needs and make necessary adjustments.

- ➢ Stay Informed: Keep up-to-date with new dietary recommendations and guidelines for CKD, and be open to modifying the diet as needed.

12. Lifestyle Considerations

Guideline: A healthy lifestyle, including regular physical activity, can complement dietary management and improve overall well-being.

Recommendation:

- ➢ Exercise: Engage in regular physical activity as recommended by a healthcare provider, which can help maintain muscle mass, control weight, and improve mood.

- ➢ Smoking and Alcohol: Avoid smoking and limit alcohol intake, as these can further strain the kidneys and exacerbate CKD symptoms.

SIMPLE AND HEALTHY KIDNEY FRIENDLY FOOD LIST FOR SENIORS WITH STAGE 4 CKD

Low Sodium food list

Vegetables

1. Cabbage
   - Serving Size: 1 cup, chopped (89g)
   - Sodium: 13 mg
   - Calories: 22 kcal
   - Nutritional Information: 5g carbohydrates, 2g dietary fiber, 1g protein, 32 mg potassium, 11 mg phosphorus
   - Medical Endorsement: Cabbage is low in potassium and sodium, making it ideal for a kidney-friendly diet.
   - Evidence-Based Recommendations: Cabbage is rich in vitamins K and C, which support overall health without overloading the kidneys.

2. Cauliflower
   - Serving Size: 1 cup, chopped (107g)
   - Sodium: 19 mg
   - Calories: 27 kcal

- Nutritional Information: 5g carbohydrates, 2g dietary fiber, 2g protein, 176 mg potassium, 40 mg phosphorus
- Medical Endorsement: Cauliflower is low in sodium and can be used as a substitute for higher potassium vegetables.
- Evidence-Based Recommendations: Cauliflower contains antioxidants and anti-inflammatory compounds that are beneficial for kidney health.

3. Bell Peppers (Green)
- Serving Size: 1 cup, sliced (92g)
- Sodium: 2 mg
- Calories: 18 kcal
- Nutritional Information: 4g carbohydrates, 1g dietary fiber, 0.6g protein, 119 mg potassium, 15 mg phosphorus
- Medical Endorsement: Bell peppers are low in potassium and sodium, making them an excellent choice for stage 4 CKD patients.
- Evidence-Based Recommendations: Rich in vitamins A and C, green bell peppers are great for enhancing immunity without stressing the kidneys.

4. Asparagus
- Serving Size: 1 cup, cooked (180g)
- Sodium: 3 mg
- Calories: 40 kcal
- Nutritional Information: 7g carbohydrates, 4g dietary fiber, 4g protein, 288 mg potassium, 65 mg phosphorus
- Medical Endorsement: Asparagus is low in sodium and contains compounds that help detoxify the kidneys.
- Evidence-Based Recommendations: It is also a good source of folate and vitamin K, supporting overall health.

5. Zucchini
- Serving Size: 1 cup, sliced (124g)
- Sodium: 6 mg
- Calories: 21 kcal
- Nutritional Information: 4g carbohydrates, 1g dietary fiber, 1g protein, 325 mg potassium, 29 mg phosphorus
- Medical Endorsement: Zucchini is a low-sodium vegetable that can be included regularly in a CKD diet.
- Evidence-Based Recommendations: High in antioxidants, zucchini helps reduce oxidative stress, which is beneficial for kidney health.

6. Radishes
- Serving Size: 1 cup, sliced (116g)
- Sodium: 45 mg
- Calories: 19 kcal
- Nutritional Information: 4g carbohydrates, 2g dietary fiber, 1g protein, 270 mg potassium, 27 mg phosphorus
- Medical Endorsement: Radishes are low in both potassium and sodium, making them a good choice for kidney patients.
- Evidence-Based Recommendations: Radishes are rich in antioxidants and support digestion, which is helpful for overall kidney function.

7. Cucumber
- Serving Size: 1 cup, sliced (119g)
- Sodium: 2 mg
- Calories: 16 kcal
- Nutritional Information: 4g carbohydrates, 1g dietary fiber, 0.7g protein, 193 mg potassium, 24 mg phosphorus
- Medical Endorsement: Cucumber is low in sodium and hydrates the body, which is crucial for kidney health.
- Evidence-Based Recommendations: Its high water content helps in flushing out toxins, supporting kidney function.

8. Lettuce (Iceberg)
- Serving Size: 1 cup, shredded (72g)
- Sodium: 10 mg
- Calories: 10 kcal
- Nutritional Information: 2g carbohydrates, 1g dietary fiber, 0.6g protein, 102 mg potassium, 7 mg phosphorus
- Medical Endorsement: Iceberg lettuce is very low in sodium and potassium, making it ideal for a renal diet.
- Evidence-Based Recommendations: Although lower in nutrients compared to other greens, it's safe and can be part of a balanced diet.

9. Turnips
- Serving Size: 1 cup, cubed (130g)
- Sodium: 87 mg
- Calories: 36 kcal
- Nutritional Information: 8g carbohydrates, 3g dietary fiber, 1g protein, 138 mg potassium, 37 mg phosphorus
- Medical Endorsement: Turnips are low in sodium and provide fiber, which is important for digestive health.
- Evidence-Based Recommendations: They can be a good alternative to potatoes for a kidney-friendly diet.

10. Carrots

- Serving Size: 1 cup, chopped (128g)
- Sodium: 88 mg
- Calories: 52 kcal
- Nutritional Information: 12g carbohydrates, 3.6g dietary fiber, 1g protein, 410 mg potassium, 35 mg phosphorus
- Medical Endorsement: Carrots are slightly higher in potassium but still manageable in controlled portions.
- Evidence-Based Recommendations: They are rich in beta-carotene, which supports eye health and overall immunity.

11. Eggplant

- Serving Size: 1 cup, cooked (99g)
- Sodium: 2 mg
- Calories: 20 kcal
- Nutritional Information: 5g carbohydrates, 2.5g dietary fiber, 0.8g protein, 188 mg potassium, 15 mg phosphorus
- Medical Endorsement: Eggplant is low in sodium and a versatile vegetable suitable for a renal diet.
- Evidence-Based Recommendations: It's a good source of fiber and can be used in various kidney-friendly recipes.

12. Green Beans
  - Serving Size: 1 cup, cooked (125g)
  - Sodium: 6 mg
  - Calories: 44 kcal
  - Nutritional Information: 10g carbohydrates, 4g dietary fiber, 2g protein, 183 mg potassium, 38 mg phosphorus
  - Medical Endorsement: Green beans are low in sodium and potassium, making them suitable for a CKD diet.
  - Evidence-Based Recommendations: They provide a good source of vitamins C and K, supporting overall health.

13. Onions
  - Serving Size: 1 cup, chopped (160g)
  - Sodium: 4 mg
  - Calories: 64 kcal
  - Nutritional Information: 15g carbohydrates, 3g dietary fiber, 1.7g protein, 234 mg potassium, 35 mg phosphorus
  - Medical Endorsement: Onions are low in sodium and can add flavor to dishes without adding salt.
  - Evidence-Based Recommendations: They contain quercetin, an antioxidant that helps reduce inflammation and protect the kidneys.

14. Summer Squash
  - Serving Size: 1 cup, sliced (130g)
  - Sodium: 4 mg
  - Calories: 18 kcal
  - Nutritional Information: 4g carbohydrates, 1g dietary fiber, 1g protein, 173 mg potassium, 30 mg phosphorus
  - Medical Endorsement: Summer squash is low in sodium and potassium, suitable for a kidney-friendly diet.
  - Evidence-Based Recommendations: It is light and easy to digest, making it ideal for seniors with CKD.

15. Kale
  - Serving Size: 1 cup, chopped (67g)
  - Sodium: 30 mg
  - Calories: 33 kcal
  - Nutritional Information: 7g carbohydrates, 1g dietary fiber, 2g protein, 329 mg potassium, 29 mg phosphorus
  - Medical Endorsement: Kale is higher in potassium but can be consumed in moderation in a renal diet.
  - Evidence-Based Recommendations: Rich in vitamins A, C, and K, kale is a nutritious vegetable that can be part of a balanced CKD diet when managed carefully.

16. Brussels Sprouts
- Serving Size: 1 cup, cooked (156g)
- Sodium: 28 mg
- Calories: 56 kcal
- Nutritional Information: 11g carbohydrates, 4g dietary fiber, 4g protein, 342 mg potassium, 64 mg phosphorus
- Medical Endorsement: Brussels sprouts are slightly higher in potassium and phosphorus, so portion control is key.
- Evidence-Based Recommendations: They are high in fiber and support digestive health, making them a beneficial choice for a CKD diet.

17. Alfalfa Sprouts
- Serving Size: 1 cup (33g)
- Sodium: 6 mg
- Calories: 8 kcal
- Nutritional Information: 1g carbohydrates, 1g dietary fiber, 1g protein, 26 mg potassium, 11 mg phosphorus
- Medical Endorsement: Alfalfa sprouts are low in sodium and can be used to add crunch to meals.
- Evidence-Based Recommendations: They are light and nutritious, making them suitable for a renal diet.

18. Rutabaga
- Serving Size: 1 cup, cubed (170g)
- Sodium: 33 mg
- Calories: 50 kcal
- Nutritional Information: 11g carbohydrates, 3g dietary fiber, 1g protein, 583 mg potassium, 53 mg phosphorus
- Medical Endorsement: Rutabaga is slightly higher in potassium, so it should be consumed in moderation.
- Evidence-Based Recommendations: It is a good source of vitamin C and fiber, supporting immune function and digestion.

19. Parsley
- Serving Size: 1/4 cup, chopped (15g)
- Sodium: 6 mg
- Calories: 4 kcal
- Nutritional Information: 1g carbohydrates, 0.5g dietary fiber, 0.5g protein, 83 mg potassium, 9 mg phosphorus
- Medical Endorsement: Parsley is low in sodium and can be used to flavor food without adding salt.
- Evidence-Based Recommendations: It has diuretic properties, which can help with fluid management in CKD.

20. Bamboo Shoots
- Serving Size: 1 cup, sliced (120g)
- Sodium: 5 mg
- Calories: 13 kcal
- Nutritional Information: 2g carbohydrates, 1g dietary fiber, 1g protein, 140 mg potassium, 11 mg phosphorus
- Medical Endorsement: Bamboo shoots are low in sodium and calories, making them a good choice for a kidney-friendly diet.
- Evidence-Based Recommendations: They are low in fat and contain fiber, aiding in digestion and overall kidney health.

1. White Rice
   - Serving Size: 1 cup, cooked (158g)
   - Sodium: 0 mg
   - Calories: 205 kcal
   - Nutritional Information: 45g carbohydrates, 0.6g dietary fiber, 4g protein, 55 mg potassium, 68 mg phosphorus
   - Medical Endorsement: White rice is a low-sodium, low-potassium grain that can be easily included in a kidney-friendly diet.
   - Evidence-Based Recommendations: It provides energy without overloading the kidneys with potassium or phosphorus.

2. Quinoa
   - Serving Size: 1 cup, cooked (185g)
   - Sodium: 13 mg
   - Calories: 222 kcal
   - Nutritional Information: 39g carbohydrates, 5g dietary fiber, 8g protein, 318 mg potassium, 281 mg phosphorus
   - Medical Endorsement: Quinoa is higher in phosphorus, so it should be

consumed in moderation, but it's also a complete protein, which is beneficial.

- Evidence-Based Recommendations: Quinoa is rich in fiber and protein, making it a nutritious option when balanced within dietary limits.

3. Couscous

- Serving Size: 1 cup, cooked (157g)
- Sodium: 8 mg
- Calories: 176 kcal
- Nutritional Information: 36g carbohydrates, 2.2g dietary fiber, 6g protein, 91 mg potassium, 48 mg phosphorus
- Medical Endorsement: Couscous is low in sodium and can be a good alternative to rice or pasta.
- Evidence-Based Recommendations: It is easy to digest and versatile, making it suitable for a kidney-friendly diet.

4. Oatmeal

- Serving Size: 1 cup, cooked (234g)
- Sodium: 2 mg
- Calories: 154 kcal
- Nutritional Information: 27g carbohydrates, 4g dietary fiber, 6g protein, 164 mg potassium, 180 mg phosphorus

- Medical Endorsement: Oatmeal is a low-sodium option, but its potassium and phosphorus content means it should be eaten in moderation.
- Evidence-Based Recommendations: Rich in fiber, oatmeal supports heart health and digestive function, which is beneficial for CKD patients.

5. Barley
- Serving Size: 1 cup, cooked (157g)
- Sodium: 6 mg
- Calories: 193 kcal
- Nutritional Information: 44g carbohydrates, 6g dietary fiber, 4g protein, 179 mg potassium, 85 mg phosphorus
- Medical Endorsement: Barley is a good source of fiber and low in sodium, making it a suitable grain for a kidney-friendly diet.
- Evidence-Based Recommendations: It has a lower glycemic index, which helps manage blood sugar levels.

6. Brown Rice
- Serving Size: 1 cup, cooked (202g)
- Sodium: 10 mg
- Calories: 216 kcal
- Nutritional Information: 45g carbohydrates, 3.5g dietary fiber, 5g

protein, 154 mg potassium, 150 mg phosphorus
- Medical Endorsement: Brown rice is slightly higher in potassium and phosphorus but is still a good source of fiber and nutrients.
- Evidence-Based Recommendations: Brown rice supports digestive health and provides steady energy, making it a good option when portioned carefully.

7. Bulgur
- Serving Size: 1 cup, cooked (182g)
- Sodium: 9 mg
- Calories: 151 kcal
- Nutritional Information: 34g carbohydrates, 8g dietary fiber, 6g protein, 62 mg potassium, 62 mg phosphorus
- Medical Endorsement: Bulgur is low in sodium and a good source of fiber, which is important for digestive health.
- Evidence-Based Recommendations: Its low potassium and phosphorus content make it safer for kidney disease patients.

8. Farro
- Serving Size: 1 cup, cooked (171g)
- Sodium: 8 mg
- Calories: 200 kcal

- Nutritional Information: 42g carbohydrates, 5g dietary fiber, 7g protein, 142 mg potassium, 115 mg phosphorus
- Medical Endorsement: Farro is low in sodium and provides a good balance of fiber and protein.
- Evidence-Based Recommendations: It's a nutrient-dense grain that supports overall health while fitting into a kidney-friendly diet when portioned properly.

9. Millet

- Serving Size: 1 cup, cooked (174g)
- Sodium: 4 mg
- Calories: 207 kcal
- Nutritional Information: 41g carbohydrates, 2.3g dietary fiber, 6g protein, 108 mg potassium, 119 mg phosphorus
- Medical Endorsement: Millet is a low-sodium, low-potassium grain, making it a good option for CKD patients.
- Evidence-Based Recommendations: It's gluten-free and can be a good alternative to other grains.

10. Polenta (Cornmeal)
   - Serving Size: 1 cup, cooked (245g)
   - Sodium: 1 mg
   - Calories: 156 kcal
   - Nutritional Information: 32g carbohydrates, 1g dietary fiber, 3g protein, 77 mg potassium, 31 mg phosphorus
   - Medical Endorsement: Polenta is low in sodium and potassium, making it kidney-friendly.
   - Evidence-Based Recommendations: It's a versatile grain that can be used as a base for many meals.

11. Wild Rice
   - Serving Size: 1 cup, cooked (164g)
   - Sodium: 5 mg
   - Calories: 166 kcal
   - Nutritional Information: 35g carbohydrates, 3g dietary fiber, 7g protein, 166 mg potassium, 134 mg phosphorus
   - Medical Endorsement: Wild rice is a good source of protein and fiber, with low sodium content.
   - Evidence-Based Recommendations: It's nutrient-dense and provides a variety of minerals, which are beneficial for seniors with CKD when portioned appropriately.

12. Amaranth
  - Serving Size: 1 cup, cooked (246g)
  - Sodium: 15 mg
  - Calories: 251 kcal
  - Nutritional Information: 46g carbohydrates, 5g dietary fiber, 9g protein, 332 mg potassium, 364 mg phosphorus
  - Medical Endorsement: Amaranth is higher in potassium and phosphorus, so it should be consumed in smaller portions.
  - Evidence-Based Recommendations: Rich in protein and fiber, amaranth can be a nutritious addition when managed carefully within a CKD diet.

13. Teff
  - Serving Size: 1 cup, cooked (252g)
  - Sodium: 7 mg
  - Calories: 255 kcal
  - Nutritional Information: 50g carbohydrates, 7g dietary fiber, 10g protein, 252 mg potassium, 231 mg phosphorus
  - Medical Endorsement: Teff is high in protein and fiber but should be consumed in moderation due to its potassium and phosphorus content.
  - Evidence-Based Recommendations: It's a nutrient-rich grain that can support

overall health when portioned appropriately.

14. Pearl Barley
  - Serving Size: 1 cup, cooked (157g)
  - Sodium: 6 mg
  - Calories: 193 kcal
  - Nutritional Information: 44g carbohydrates, 6g dietary fiber, 4g protein, 179 mg potassium, 85 mg phosphorus
  - Medical Endorsement: Pearl barley is low in sodium and provides dietary fiber, beneficial for digestion.
  - Evidence-Based Recommendations: It has a lower glycemic index, making it a good choice for managing blood sugar levels.

15. Buckwheat
  - Serving Size: 1 cup, cooked (168g)
  - Sodium: 5 mg
  - Calories: 155 kcal
  - Nutritional Information: 33g carbohydrates, 5g dietary fiber, 6g protein, 150 mg potassium, 115 mg phosphorus
  - Medical Endorsement: Buckwheat is low in sodium and is gluten-free, making it suitable for those with sensitivities.

- Evidence-Based Recommendations: It's rich in nutrients and supports heart health, which is important for CKD patients.

Snacks

1. Unsalted Rice Cakes
   - Serving Size: 1 rice cake (9g)
   - Sodium: 0 mg
   - Calories: 35 kcal
   - Nutritional Information: 7g carbohydrates, 0g dietary fiber, 1g protein, 10 mg potassium, 15 mg phosphorus
   - Medical Endorsement: Unsalted rice cakes are low in sodium and can be topped with low-sodium spreads or vegetables.
   - Evidence-Based Recommendations: A light, crunchy snack that can be paired with other kidney-friendly toppings.

2. Apple Slices with Unsalted Almond Butter
   - Serving Size: 1 medium apple with 1 tbsp unsalted almond butter (150g total)
   - Sodium: 1 mg
   - Calories: 140 kcal
   - Nutritional Information: 20g carbohydrates, 4g dietary fiber, 3g

protein, 200 mg potassium, 40 mg phosphorus
- Medical Endorsement: Apples are low in potassium and sodium, and almond butter provides healthy fats with minimal sodium.
- Evidence-Based Recommendations: A balanced snack that offers fiber and protein while being gentle on the kidneys.

3. Unsalted Popcorn

- Serving Size: 3 cups, air-popped (24g)
- Sodium: 1 mg
- Calories: 93 kcal
- Nutritional Information: 18g carbohydrates, 3.6g dietary fiber, 3g protein, 69 mg potassium, 58 mg phosphorus
- Medical Endorsement: Air-popped popcorn without added salt is a kidney-friendly, low-sodium snack.
- Evidence-Based Recommendations: Popcorn is a whole grain that provides fiber and satisfies cravings for a crunchy snack.

4. Fresh Blueberries

- Serving Size: 1 cup (148g)
- Sodium: 1 mg
- Calories: 84 kcal

- Nutritional Information: 21g carbohydrates, 4g dietary fiber, 1g protein, 114 mg potassium, 18 mg phosphorus
- Medical Endorsement: Blueberries are low in sodium, potassium, and phosphorus, making them an excellent fruit choice.
- Evidence-Based Recommendations: Rich in antioxidants, blueberries support overall health and can be enjoyed alone or with other snacks.

5. Celery Sticks with Cream Cheese
- Serving Size: 1 large stalk with 1 tbsp cream cheese (50g total)
- Sodium: 40 mg
- Calories: 50 kcal
- Nutritional Information: 3g carbohydrates, 1g dietary fiber, 1g protein, 150 mg potassium, 40 mg phosphorus
- Medical Endorsement: Celery is low in sodium, and cream cheese can be chosen in a low-sodium variety to keep the snack kidney-friendly.
- Evidence-Based Recommendations: This snack is easy to prepare and offers a crunchy, creamy texture combination.

6. Strawberries
- Serving Size: 1 cup, sliced (166g)
- Sodium: 1 mg
- Calories: 53 kcal
- Nutritional Information: 13g carbohydrates, 3g dietary fiber, 1g protein, 254 mg potassium, 23 mg phosphorus
- Medical Endorsement: Strawberries are low in sodium and provide vitamins and antioxidants that support kidney health.
- Evidence-Based Recommendations: They can be eaten fresh or added to other snacks for a sweet, nutritious boost.

7. Cucumber Slices with Hummus
- Serving Size: 1/2 cup cucumber slices with 2 tbsp low-sodium hummus (150g total)
- Sodium: 50 mg
- Calories: 70 kcal
- Nutritional Information: 8g carbohydrates, 2g dietary fiber, 2g protein, 150 mg potassium, 40 mg phosphorus
- Medical Endorsement: Cucumber is low in potassium and sodium, and choosing a low-sodium hummus makes this snack kidney-friendly.

- Evidence-Based Recommendations: Provides hydration and nutrients without excessive sodium, ideal for CKD patients.

8. Pineapple Chunks
   - Serving Size: 1 cup, chunks (165g)
   - Sodium: 2 mg
   - Calories: 82 kcal
   - Nutritional Information: 21g carbohydrates, 2g dietary fiber, 1g protein, 180 mg potassium, 13 mg phosphorus
   - Medical Endorsement: Pineapple is low in sodium and potassium, making it a safe fruit choice for those with CKD.
   - Evidence-Based Recommendations: It's a refreshing and sweet snack that can be enjoyed on its own or in fruit salads.

9. Graham Crackers
   - Serving Size: 2 crackers (14g)
   - Sodium: 35 mg
   - Calories: 59 kcal
   - Nutritional Information: 11g carbohydrates, 0.5g dietary fiber, 1g protein, 35 mg potassium, 11 mg phosphorus
   - Medical Endorsement: Graham crackers are low in sodium and provide a light, sweet snack option.

- Evidence-Based Recommendations: They can be enjoyed with fruit or on their own as a quick snack.

10. Unsalted Pumpkin Seeds
    - Serving Size: 1 ounce (28g)
    - Sodium: 5 mg
    - Calories: 151 kcal
    - Nutritional Information: 5g carbohydrates, 1g dietary fiber, 7g protein, 226 mg potassium, 294 mg phosphorus
    - Medical Endorsement: Pumpkin seeds are higher in potassium and phosphorus, so they should be consumed in moderation.
    - Evidence-Based Recommendations: They provide healthy fats and protein, making them a nutritious snack when portioned properly.

11. Rice Crackers
    - Serving Size: 10 crackers (20g)
    - Sodium: 20 mg
    - Calories: 70 kcal
    - Nutritional Information: 15g carbohydrates, 0g dietary fiber, 1g protein, 30 mg potassium, 20 mg phosphorus

- Medical Endorsement: Rice crackers are low in sodium and can be enjoyed as a light, crunchy snack.
- Evidence-Based Recommendations: Pair with kidney-friendly toppings like cucumber or low-sodium cheese for added flavor.

12. Peach Slices

- Serving Size: 1 medium peach (150g)
- Sodium: 0 mg
- Calories: 58 kcal
- Nutritional Information: 14g carbohydrates, 2g dietary fiber, 1g protein, 285 mg potassium, 19 mg phosphorus
- Medical Endorsement: Peaches are low in sodium and provide vitamins and fiber, making them a good snack option.
- Evidence-Based Recommendations: Enjoy fresh peach slices on their own or with a dollop of whipped cream for a simple treat.

13. Unsalted Almonds

- Serving Size: 1 ounce (28g)
- Sodium: 1 mg
- Calories: 160 kcal
- Nutritional Information: 6g carbohydrates, 3.5g dietary fiber, 6g

protein, 200 mg potassium, 150 mg phosphorus
- Medical Endorsement: Unsalted almonds are high in potassium and phosphorus, so portion control is important.
- Evidence-Based Recommendations: A good source of healthy fats and protein, they can be a nutritious part of a kidney-friendly diet when eaten in moderation.

14. Melon Cubes (Honeydew or Cantaloupe)
- Serving Size: 1 cup, cubed (170g)
- Sodium: 25 mg
- Calories: 60 kcal
- Nutritional Information: 15g carbohydrates, 1.5g dietary fiber, 1g protein, 388 mg potassium, 15 mg phosphorus
- Medical Endorsement: Melons are higher in potassium, so they should be eaten in moderation, but they are low in sodium.
- Evidence-Based Recommendations: Melons are hydrating and refreshing, making them a great choice for a light snack.

15. Rice Pudding
- Serving Size: 1/2 cup (142g)
- Sodium: 40 mg
- Calories: 130 kcal
- Nutritional Information: 22g carbohydrates, 0.5g dietary fiber, 3g protein, 130 mg potassium, 100 mg phosphorus
- Medical Endorsement: Rice pudding is a kidney-friendly dessert option when prepared with low-sodium ingredients.
- Evidence-Based Recommendations: Enjoy as a sweet treat that fits within dietary sodium and phosphorus guidelines.

Fruits

1. Apples
- Serving Size: 1 medium apple (182g)
- Sodium: 1 mg
- Calories: 95 kcal
- Nutritional Information: 25g carbohydrates, 4g dietary fiber, 0.5g protein, 195 mg potassium, 20 mg phosphorus
- Medical Endorsement: Apples are low in sodium and provide fiber and antioxidants, which are beneficial for overall health.

- Evidence-Based Recommendations: Ideal for snacking or adding to salads, apples are safe and kidney-friendly.

2. Blueberries
- Serving Size: 1 cup (148g)
- Sodium: 1 mg
- Calories: 84 kcal
- Nutritional Information: 21g carbohydrates, 4g dietary fiber, 1g protein, 114 mg potassium, 18 mg phosphorus
- Medical Endorsement: Blueberries are rich in antioxidants and low in potassium, phosphorus, and sodium.
- Evidence-Based Recommendations: Enjoy them fresh or added to cereal or yogurt for a nutritious snack.

3. Strawberries
- Serving Size: 1 cup, sliced (166g)
- Sodium: 1 mg
- Calories: 53 kcal
- Nutritional Information: 13g carbohydrates, 3g dietary fiber, 1g protein, 254 mg potassium, 23 mg phosphorus
- Medical Endorsement: Strawberries are low in sodium and packed with vitamins, making them a heart-healthy choice.

- Evidence-Based Recommendations: Versatile and easy to include in many meals, from breakfasts to desserts.

4. Grapes
- Serving Size: 1 cup (151g)
- Sodium: 2 mg
- Calories: 104 kcal
- Nutritional Information: 27g carbohydrates, 1.4g dietary fiber, 1g protein, 288 mg potassium, 30 mg phosphorus
- Medical Endorsement: Grapes are hydrating and low in sodium, with a moderate amount of potassium.
- Evidence-Based Recommendations: They can be eaten fresh, frozen, or as a sweet addition to salads.

5. Peaches
- Serving Size: 1 medium peach (150g)
- Sodium: 0 mg
- Calories: 58 kcal
- Nutritional Information: 14g carbohydrates, 2g dietary fiber, 1g protein, 285 mg potassium, 19 mg phosphorus
- Medical Endorsement: Peaches are low in sodium and provide vitamins A and C.

- Evidence-Based Recommendations: Great for eating fresh, in smoothies, or as part of a fruit salad.

6. Pineapple
- Serving Size: 1 cup, chunks (165g)
- Sodium: 2 mg
- Calories: 82 kcal
- Nutritional Information: 21g carbohydrates, 2g dietary fiber, 1g protein, 180 mg potassium, 13 mg phosphorus
- Medical Endorsement: Pineapple is low in sodium and provides a good source of vitamin C.
- Evidence-Based Recommendations: Pineapple can be enjoyed fresh, grilled, or as a topping for dishes.

7. Watermelon
- Serving Size: 1 cup, diced (152g)
- Sodium: 2 mg
- Calories: 46 kcal
- Nutritional Information: 12g carbohydrates, 0.6g dietary fiber, 1g protein, 170 mg potassium, 11 mg phosphorus
- Medical Endorsement: Watermelon is hydrating and low in sodium, with moderate potassium content.

- Evidence-Based Recommendations: Ideal for a refreshing snack or dessert, especially in hot weather.

8. Cranberries

- Serving Size: 1/2 cup, fresh (50g)
- Sodium: 1 mg
- Calories: 25 kcal
- Nutritional Information: 6g carbohydrates, 2g dietary fiber, 0.2g protein, 44 mg potassium, 6 mg phosphorus
- Medical Endorsement: Cranberries are low in sodium and potassium and are known for supporting urinary tract health.
- Evidence-Based Recommendations: Enjoy them fresh, dried (unsweetened), or in sauces.

9. Raspberries

- Serving Size: 1 cup (123g)
- Sodium: 1 mg
- Calories: 64 kcal
- Nutritional Information: 15g carbohydrates, 8g dietary fiber, 1.5g protein, 186 mg potassium, 29 mg phosphorus
- Medical Endorsement: Raspberries are high in fiber and low in sodium, potassium, and phosphorus.

- Evidence-Based Recommendations: They're perfect for snacking or adding to desserts, salads, or smoothies.

10. Tangerines
    - Serving Size: 1 medium tangerine (109g)
    - Sodium: 2 mg
    - Calories: 50 kcal
    - Nutritional Information: 13g carbohydrates, 1.6g dietary fiber, 0.8g protein, 132 mg potassium, 20 mg phosphorus
    - Medical Endorsement: Tangerines are low in sodium and provide a good source of vitamin C.
    - Evidence-Based Recommendations: A convenient, portable snack that's easy to include in a kidney-friendly diet.

11. Plums
    - Serving Size: 1 medium plum (66g)
    - Sodium: 0 mg
    - Calories: 30 kcal
    - Nutritional Information: 8g carbohydrates, 1g dietary fiber, 0.5g protein, 104 mg potassium, 11 mg phosphorus
    - Medical Endorsement: Plums are low in sodium and moderate in potassium,

making them a safe option for CKD patients.
- Evidence-Based Recommendations: Enjoy fresh or as part of a fruit salad for a sweet, kidney-friendly snack.

12. Cantaloupe
- Serving Size: 1 cup, diced (160g)
- Sodium: 28 mg
- Calories: 53 kcal
- Nutritional Information: 13g carbohydrates, 1.4g dietary fiber, 1.3g protein, 427 mg potassium, 17 mg phosphorus
- Medical Endorsement: Cantaloupe is low in sodium, but higher in potassium, so it should be consumed in moderation.
- Evidence-Based Recommendations: It's hydrating and refreshing, perfect for a light snack or dessert.

13. Cherries
- Serving Size: 1 cup (138g)
- Sodium: 0 mg
- Calories: 87 kcal
- Nutritional Information: 22g carbohydrates, 3g dietary fiber, 1.5g protein, 306 mg potassium, 21 mg phosphorus

- Medical Endorsement: Cherries are low in sodium and provide antioxidants that are beneficial for kidney health.
- Evidence-Based Recommendations: Eat them fresh as a snack or add to desserts and salads.

14. Mango

- Serving Size: 1/2 cup, sliced (83g)
- Sodium: 1 mg
- Calories: 50 kcal
- Nutritional Information: 13g carbohydrates, 1.6g dietary fiber, 0.4g protein, 135 mg potassium, 10 mg phosphorus
- Medical Endorsement: Mango is low in sodium and provides vitamins A and C, which are important for overall health.
- Evidence-Based Recommendations: Enjoy in moderation, fresh, or in smoothies, for a tropical treat.

15. Pears

- Serving Size: 1 medium pear (178g)
- Sodium: 2 mg
- Calories: 101 kcal
- Nutritional Information: 27g carbohydrates, 6g dietary fiber, 1g protein, 206 mg potassium, 20 mg phosphorus

- Medical Endorsement: Pears are low in sodium and provide fiber, which supports digestive health.
- Evidence-Based Recommendations: Enjoy fresh or poached as part of a kidney-friendly diet.

Proteins

1. Skinless Chicken Breast
   - Serving Size: 3 ounces (85g)
   - Sodium: 60 mg
   - Calories: 140 kcal
   - Nutritional Information: 26g protein, 0g carbohydrates, 1g fat, 300 mg potassium, 220 mg phosphorus
   - Medical Endorsement: Skinless chicken breast is a lean source of protein with low sodium when not processed or seasoned.
   - Evidence-Based Recommendations: Excellent choice for a low-sodium, high-protein diet. Cook without added salt.

2. Egg Whites
   - Serving Size: 1 large egg white (33g)
   - Sodium: 55 mg
   - Calories: 17 kcal

- Nutritional Information: 4g protein, 0g carbohydrates, 0g fat, 54 mg potassium, 5 mg phosphorus
- Medical Endorsement: Egg whites are a high-quality protein source with minimal sodium and phosphorus.
- Evidence-Based Recommendations: Suitable for making omelets or adding to recipes for added protein without excess sodium.

3. Tofu (Firm, Light)

- Serving Size: 1/2 cup (124g)
- Sodium: 8 mg
- Calories: 94 kcal
- Nutritional Information: 10g protein, 2g carbohydrates, 5g fat, 150 mg potassium, 100 mg phosphorus
- Medical Endorsement: Tofu is a good plant-based protein option with low sodium and can be a versatile ingredient.
- Evidence-Based Recommendations: Ideal for stir-fries, soups, or salads. Choose low-sodium varieties if available.

4. Lean Ground Turkey

- Serving Size: 3 ounces (85g)
- Sodium: 70 mg
- Calories: 150 kcal

- Nutritional Information: 22g protein, 0g carbohydrates, 7g fat, 300 mg potassium, 240 mg phosphorus
- Medical Endorsement: Lean ground turkey is a lower-fat alternative to beef and has less sodium if not processed.
- Evidence-Based Recommendations: Use in recipes like burgers or meatloaf without added salt or sodium-containing ingredients.

5. Cod (Baked)

- Serving Size: 3 ounces (85g)
- Sodium: 60 mg
- Calories: 70 kcal
- Nutritional Information: 15g protein, 0g carbohydrates, 0.5g fat, 300 mg potassium, 200 mg phosphorus
- Medical Endorsement: Cod is a lean fish with low sodium and phosphorus, making it suitable for CKD diets.
- Evidence-Based Recommendations: Bake or grill with kidney-friendly herbs and spices.

6. Lentils (Boiled)

- Serving Size: 1/2 cup (99g)
- Sodium: 1 mg
- Calories: 115 kcal

- Nutritional Information: 9g protein, 20g carbohydrates, 0.4g fat, 365 mg potassium, 95 mg phosphorus
- Medical Endorsement: Lentils are a good plant-based protein but should be consumed in moderation due to potassium and phosphorus.
- Evidence-Based Recommendations: Incorporate in small amounts into soups, stews, or salads.

7. Greek Yogurt (Plain, Non-Fat)

- Serving Size: 1/2 cup (130g)
- Sodium: 60 mg
- Calories: 80 kcal
- Nutritional Information: 10g protein, 6g carbohydrates, 0g fat, 150 mg potassium, 90 mg phosphorus
- Medical Endorsement: Plain Greek yogurt is high in protein and relatively low in sodium, beneficial for kidney diets.
- Evidence-Based Recommendations: Use as a snack or in smoothies. Avoid flavored varieties which may have added sodium or sugar.

8. Quinoa (Cooked)

- Serving Size: 1/2 cup (92g)
- Sodium: 7 mg
- Calories: 111 kcal

- Nutritional Information: 4g protein, 19g carbohydrates, 2g fat, 118 mg potassium, 29 mg phosphorus
- Medical Endorsement: Quinoa is a complete protein source with low sodium and moderate potassium.
- Evidence-Based Recommendations: Use as a base for salads or side dishes, ensuring to control portion sizes due to potassium content.

9. Edamame (Shelled, Cooked)

- Serving Size: 1/2 cup (78g)
- Sodium: 0 mg
- Calories: 120 kcal
- Nutritional Information: 11g protein, 10g carbohydrates, 5g fat, 300 mg potassium, 90 mg phosphorus
- Medical Endorsement: Edamame provides plant-based protein with low sodium. However, it is higher in potassium.
- Evidence-Based Recommendations: Enjoy in moderation, focusing on portion control.

10. Cottage Cheese (Low-Sodium)

- Serving Size: 1/2 cup (113g)
- Sodium: 370 mg
- Calories: 90 kcal

- Nutritional Information: 12g protein, 4g carbohydrates, 1g fat, 200 mg potassium, 200 mg phosphorus
- Medical Endorsement: Choose low-sodium varieties to minimize sodium intake while getting protein.
- Evidence-Based Recommendations: Good for snacking or adding to meals; check labels for sodium content.

11. Chicken Thigh (Skinless)

- Serving Size: 3 ounces (85g)
- Sodium: 65 mg
- Calories: 180 kcal
- Nutritional Information: 22g protein, 0g carbohydrates, 10g fat, 290 mg potassium, 210 mg phosphorus
- Medical Endorsement: Skinless chicken thighs are a more flavorful alternative to breasts with moderate sodium levels.
- Evidence-Based Recommendations: Use in various recipes, but avoid adding salt or high-sodium ingredients.

12. Turkey Breast (Cooked)

- Serving Size: 3 ounces (85g)
- Sodium: 60 mg
- Calories: 135 kcal
- Nutritional Information: 30g protein, 0g carbohydrates, 1g fat, 320 mg potassium, 220 mg phosphorus

- Medical Endorsement: Turkey breast is a lean, high-protein option with low sodium when unprocessed.
- Evidence-Based Recommendations: Roast or grill and use in sandwiches or salads.

13. White Fish (Like Haddock, Baked)
  - Serving Size: 3 ounces (85g)
  - Sodium: 50 mg
  - Calories: 70 kcal
  - Nutritional Information: 15g protein, 0g carbohydrates, 0.5g fat, 280 mg potassium, 180 mg phosphorus
  - Medical Endorsement: White fish is low in sodium and phosphorus, making it suitable for a kidney-friendly diet.
  - Evidence-Based Recommendations: Opt for fresh or frozen, avoiding pre-seasoned or processed varieties.

14. Chickpeas (Boiled)
  - Serving Size: 1/2 cup (82g)
  - Sodium: 6 mg
  - Calories: 135 kcal
  - Nutritional Information: 7g protein, 22g carbohydrates, 2g fat, 238 mg potassium, 90 mg phosphorus
  - Medical Endorsement: Chickpeas are a good plant-based protein source but

should be limited due to potassium and phosphorus.
- Evidence-Based Recommendations: Use in moderation and incorporate into dishes like salads or soups.

15. Tempeh
- Serving Size: 1/2 cup (94g)
- Sodium: 7 mg
- Calories: 160 kcal
- Nutritional Information: 16g protein, 9g carbohydrates, 8g fat, 260 mg potassium, 180 mg phosphorus
- Medical Endorsement: Tempeh is a fermented soy product with a moderate amount of potassium and phosphorus, but low sodium.
- Evidence-Based Recommendations: Can be used in various dishes as a protein substitute, but monitor portion sizes.

Dairy Alternatives

1. Unsweetened Almond Milk
   - Serving Size: 1 cup (240ml)
   - Sodium: 160 mg
   - Calories: 30 kcal
   - Nutritional Information: 1g protein, 1g carbohydrates, 2.5g fat, 160 mg potassium, 50 mg phosphorus
   - Medical Endorsement: Almond milk is low in sodium and a good alternative to dairy milk. Opt for unsweetened versions to avoid added sugars.
   - Evidence-Based Recommendations: Suitable for drinking, cooking, or adding to cereals.

2. Unsweetened Coconut Milk
   - Serving Size: 1 cup (240ml)
   - Sodium: 30 mg
   - Calories: 45 kcal
   - Nutritional Information: 0g protein, 1g carbohydrates, 4.5g fat, 60 mg potassium, 22 mg phosphorus
   - Medical Endorsement: Coconut milk is low in sodium and can be a good choice for those avoiding dairy.
   - Evidence-Based Recommendations: Ideal for cooking, baking, or as a beverage.

3. Rice Milk (Unsweetened)
- Serving Size: 1 cup (240ml)
- Sodium: 80 mg
- Calories: 60 kcal
- Nutritional Information: 1g protein, 11g carbohydrates, 1g fat, 80 mg potassium, 20 mg phosphorus
- Medical Endorsement: Rice milk is low in sodium and provides a mild, neutral flavor.
- Evidence-Based Recommendations: Use in cooking, baking, or as a drink, but ensure it's unsweetened.

4. Soy Milk (Unsweetened)
- Serving Size: 1 cup (240ml)
- Sodium: 100 mg
- Calories: 80 kcal
- Nutritional Information: 7g protein, 4g carbohydrates, 4g fat, 300 mg potassium, 50 mg phosphorus
- Medical Endorsement: Soy milk is a good source of plant-based protein and is low in sodium when unsweetened.
- Evidence-Based Recommendations: Suitable for drinking or using in recipes; choose low-sodium and unsweetened varieties.

5. Hemp Milk (Unsweetened)
- Serving Size: 1 cup (240ml)
- Sodium: 140 mg
- Calories: 60 kcal
- Nutritional Information: 3g protein, 1g carbohydrates, 4.5g fat, 300 mg potassium, 30 mg phosphorus
- Medical Endorsement: Hemp milk is low in sodium and contains beneficial omega-3 fatty acids.
- Evidence-Based Recommendations: Use as a beverage or in recipes; ensure it is unsweetened.

6. Cashew Milk (Unsweetened)
- Serving Size: 1 cup (240ml)
- Sodium: 75 mg
- Calories: 25 kcal
- Nutritional Information: 1g protein, 1g carbohydrates, 2g fat, 150 mg potassium, 40 mg phosphorus
- Medical Endorsement: Cashew milk is low in sodium and provides a creamy texture without dairy.
- Evidence-Based Recommendations: Ideal for use in cooking, baking, or as a drink. Opt for unsweetened varieties.

7. Oat Milk (Unsweetened)
- Serving Size: 1 cup (240ml)
- Sodium: 90 mg
- Calories: 60 kcal
- Nutritional Information: 2g protein, 16g carbohydrates, 1.5g fat, 350 mg potassium, 30 mg phosphorus
- Medical Endorsement: Oat milk is low in sodium and provides a good source of fiber.
- Evidence-Based Recommendations: Suitable for drinking, adding to cereals, or using in recipes. Choose unsweetened versions.

8. Flax Milk (Unsweetened)
- Serving Size: 1 cup (240ml)
- Sodium: 120 mg
- Calories: 25 kcal
- Nutritional Information: 1g protein, 1g carbohydrates, 2.5g fat, 90 mg potassium, 30 mg phosphorus
- Medical Endorsement: Flax milk is low in sodium and contains omega-3 fatty acids.
- Evidence-Based Recommendations: Use in beverages, cooking, or baking. Ensure it is unsweetened.

9. Almond Milk (Vanilla, Unsweetened)
- Serving Size: 1 cup (240ml)
- Sodium: 180 mg
- Calories: 40 kcal
- Nutritional Information: 1g protein, 2g carbohydrates, 3g fat, 160 mg potassium, 55 mg phosphorus
- Medical Endorsement: Vanilla-flavored almond milk is low in sodium but may contain added sugars. Choose unsweetened varieties.
- Evidence-Based Recommendations: Use in moderation or opt for plain unsweetened versions for fewer additives.

10. Macadamia Milk (Unsweetened)
- Serving Size: 1 cup (240ml)
- Sodium: 5 mg
- Calories: 50 kcal
- Nutritional Information: 1g protein, 1g carbohydrates, 4.5g fat, 80 mg potassium, 10 mg phosphorus
- Medical Endorsement: Macadamia milk is low in sodium and has a creamy texture.
- Evidence-Based Recommendations: Ideal for beverages or cooking. Ensure it is unsweetened.

11. Pea Milk (Unsweetened)
- Serving Size: 1 cup (240ml)
- Sodium: 120 mg
- Calories: 70 kcal
- Nutritional Information: 8g protein, 3g carbohydrates, 4g fat, 270 mg potassium, 50 mg phosphorus
- Medical Endorsement: Pea milk is high in protein and low in sodium. Opt for unsweetened versions.
- Evidence-Based Recommendations: Good for drinking or adding to recipes.

12. Soy Yogurt (Unsweetened)
- Serving Size: 1/2 cup (120g)
- Sodium: 50 mg
- Calories: 80 kcal
- Nutritional Information: 6g protein, 7g carbohydrates, 4g fat, 150 mg potassium, 30 mg phosphorus
- Medical Endorsement: Soy yogurt provides protein and is lower in sodium compared to dairy yogurt.
- Evidence-Based Recommendations: Use as a snack or part of meals. Choose unsweetened varieties to avoid added sugars.

13. Coconut Yogurt (Unsweetened)
   - Serving Size: 1/2 cup (120g)
   - Sodium: 30 mg
   - Calories: 50 kcal
   - Nutritional Information: 1g protein, 6g carbohydrates, 3g fat, 100 mg potassium, 20 mg phosphorus
   - Medical Endorsement: Coconut yogurt is low in sodium and provides a dairy-free alternative with healthy fats.
   - Evidence-Based Recommendations: Suitable for snacks or incorporating into meals, choose unsweetened versions.

14. Almond-Based Cheese (Unsweetened)
   - Serving Size: 1 ounce (28g)
   - Sodium: 120 mg
   - Calories: 80 kcal
   - Nutritional Information: 3g protein, 2g carbohydrates, 6g fat, 80 mg potassium, 30 mg phosphorus
   - Medical Endorsement: Almond-based cheese offers a low-sodium alternative to traditional cheese.
   - Evidence-Based Recommendations: Use in moderation as a replacement for cheese in recipes or as a snack.

15. Cashew-Based Cheese (Unsweetened)
- Serving Size: 1 ounce (28g)
- Sodium: 100 mg
- Calories: 90 kcal
- Nutritional Information: 4g protein, 2g carbohydrates, 7g fat, 90 mg potassium, 40 mg phosphorus
- Medical Endorsement: Cashew-based cheese is low in sodium and can be a good substitute for regular cheese.
- Evidence-Based Recommendations: Suitable for incorporating into recipes or eating as a snack.

Herbs and spices

1. Basil (Fresh)
- Serving Size: 1 tablespoon (2g)
- Sodium: 0 mg
- Calories: 1 kcal
- Nutritional Information: 0g protein, 0g carbohydrates, 0g fat, 10 mg potassium, 8 mg phosphorus
- Medical Endorsement: Basil adds flavor without sodium and has antioxidants.
- Evidence-Based Recommendations: Use fresh basil in salads, sauces, and as a garnish.

2. Cilantro (Fresh)
- Serving Size: 1 tablespoon (1g)
- Sodium: 0 mg
- Calories: 0 kcal
- Nutritional Information: 0g protein, 0g carbohydrates, 0g fat, 11 mg potassium, 5 mg phosphorus
- Medical Endorsement: Cilantro is a flavorful herb with no sodium, beneficial for adding zest to dishes.
- Evidence-Based Recommendations: Use in salads, soups, or as a garnish.

3. Parsley (Fresh)
- Serving Size: 1 tablespoon (2g)
- Sodium: 0 mg
- Calories: 1 kcal
- Nutritional Information: 0g protein, 0g carbohydrates, 0g fat, 10 mg potassium, 10 mg phosphorus
- Medical Endorsement: Parsley is low in sodium and provides a fresh flavor.
- Evidence-Based Recommendations: Ideal for seasoning, garnishing, and adding to salads.

4. Rosemary (Fresh)
- Serving Size: 1 tablespoon (2g)
- Sodium: 0 mg
- Calories: 2 kcal

- Nutritional Information: 0g protein, 0g carbohydrates, 0g fat, 10 mg potassium, 8 mg phosphorus
- Medical Endorsement: Rosemary enhances flavor without adding sodium and has antioxidant properties.
- Evidence-Based Recommendations: Use in marinades, roasted dishes, and as a seasoning.

5. Thyme (Fresh)

- Serving Size: 1 tablespoon (2g)
- Sodium: 0 mg
- Calories: 2 kcal
- Nutritional Information: 0g protein, 0g carbohydrates, 0g fat, 10 mg potassium, 7 mg phosphorus
- Medical Endorsement: Thyme adds a rich flavor with no sodium and is beneficial for cooking.
- Evidence-Based Recommendations: Use in soups, stews, and as a seasoning for meats and vegetables.

6. Oregano (Dried)

- Serving Size: 1 teaspoon (1g)
- Sodium: 0 mg
- Calories: 3 kcal
- Nutritional Information: 0g protein, 1g carbohydrates, 0g fat, 15 mg potassium, 5 mg phosphorus

- Medical Endorsement: Dried oregano is a sodium-free herb that adds depth to flavors.
- Evidence-Based Recommendations: Use in sauces, marinades, and Italian dishes.

7. Dill (Fresh)
  - Serving Size: 1 tablespoon (2g)
  - Sodium: 0 mg
  - Calories: 1 kcal
  - Nutritional Information: 0g protein, 0g carbohydrates, 0g fat, 10 mg potassium, 7 mg phosphorus
  - Medical Endorsement: Dill provides flavor without sodium and has a fresh taste.
  - Evidence-Based Recommendations: Excellent for seasoning fish, vegetables, and salads.

8. Sage (Fresh)
  - Serving Size: 1 tablespoon (2g)
  - Sodium: 0 mg
  - Calories: 1 kcal
  - Nutritional Information: 0g protein, 0g carbohydrates, 0g fat, 10 mg potassium, 6 mg phosphorus
  - Medical Endorsement: Sage adds a unique flavor with no sodium and has beneficial antioxidants.

- Evidence-Based Recommendations: Use in savory dishes, stuffing, and as a seasoning.

9. Cumin (Ground)
   - Serving Size: 1 teaspoon (2g)
   - Sodium: 0 mg
   - Calories: 8 kcal
   - Nutritional Information: 0g protein, 1g carbohydrates, 0g fat, 30 mg potassium, 11 mg phosphorus
   - Medical Endorsement: Cumin is low in sodium and adds a warm, earthy flavor to dishes.
   - Evidence-Based Recommendations: Use in curries, soups, and spice blends.

10. Cinnamon (Ground)
    - Serving Size: 1 teaspoon (2g)
    - Sodium: 0 mg
    - Calories: 6 kcal
    - Nutritional Information: 0g protein, 2g carbohydrates, 0g fat, 15 mg potassium, 4 mg phosphorus
    - Medical Endorsement: Cinnamon provides flavor without sodium and has potential health benefits.
    - Evidence-Based Recommendations: Use in baking, oatmeal, and as a spice for savory dishes.

11. Paprika (Ground)
- Serving Size: 1 teaspoon (2g)
- Sodium: 0 mg
- Calories: 6 kcal
- Nutritional Information: 0g protein, 2g carbohydrates, 0g fat, 12 mg potassium, 6 mg phosphorus
- Medical Endorsement: Paprika is sodium-free and adds a mild peppery flavor.
- Evidence-Based Recommendations: Use in soups, stews, and to add color to dishes.

12. Turmeric (Ground)
- Serving Size: 1 teaspoon (2g)
- Sodium: 0 mg
- Calories: 8 kcal
- Nutritional Information: 0g protein, 2g carbohydrates, 0g fat, 40 mg potassium, 12 mg phosphorus
- Medical Endorsement: Turmeric adds color and flavor without sodium and has anti-inflammatory properties.
- Evidence-Based Recommendations: Use in curries, rice dishes, and as a color enhancer in recipes.

13. Ginger (Fresh)
- Serving Size: 1 tablespoon (6g)
- Sodium: 0 mg
- Calories: 5 kcal
- Nutritional Information: 0g protein, 1g carbohydrates, 0g fat, 25 mg potassium, 4 mg phosphorus
- Medical Endorsement: Fresh ginger provides a spicy flavor without sodium and supports digestion.
- Evidence-Based Recommendations: Use in teas, stir-fries, and marinades.

14. Garlic Powder (Unsalted)
- Serving Size: 1/4 teaspoon (1g)
- Sodium: 0 mg
- Calories: 4 kcal
- Nutritional Information: 0g protein, 1g carbohydrates, 0g fat, 10 mg potassium, 2 mg phosphorus
- Medical Endorsement: Garlic powder offers a concentrated garlic flavor without sodium.
- Evidence-Based Recommendations: Use to season meats, vegetables, and pasta dishes.

15. Chili Powder (Unsalted)
- Serving Size: 1 teaspoon (2g)
- Sodium: 0 mg
- Calories: 8 kcal

- Nutritional Information: 0g protein, 2g carbohydrates, 0g fat, 30 mg potassium, 10 mg phosphorus
- Medical Endorsement: Chili powder adds heat and flavor without sodium.
- Evidence-Based Recommendations: Use in soups, stews, and to add spiciness to dishes.

Fruits

1. Apples
- Serving Size: 1 medium apple (182g)
- Phosphorus: 20 mg
- Calories: 95 kcal
- Nutritional Information: 0.5g protein, 25g carbohydrates, 0.3g fat, 195 mg potassium
- Medical Endorsement: Apples are low in phosphorus and high in fiber.
- Evidence-Based Recommendations: Ideal for snacks or in salads. Peel the skin to reduce potassium content further.

2. Pears
- Serving Size: 1 medium pear (178g)
- Phosphorus: 20 mg
- Calories: 102 kcal
- Nutritional Information: 0.5g protein, 27g carbohydrates, 0.2g fat, 190 mg potassium
- Medical Endorsement: Pears are low in phosphorus and provide a good source of dietary fiber.

- Evidence-Based Recommendations: Consume fresh or canned in juice for a refreshing snack.

3. Peaches

- Serving Size: 1 medium peach (150g)
- Phosphorus: 18 mg
- Calories: 58 kcal
- Nutritional Information: 1g protein, 14g carbohydrates, 0.2g fat, 285 mg potassium
- Medical Endorsement: Peaches are low in phosphorus and rich in vitamins.
- Evidence-Based Recommendations: Enjoy fresh or canned without added sugars.

4. Plums

- Serving Size: 1 medium plum (66g)
- Phosphorus: 14 mg
- Calories: 30 kcal
- Nutritional Information: 0.5g protein, 8g carbohydrates, 0g fat, 113 mg potassium
- Medical Endorsement: Plums are low in phosphorus and provide antioxidants.
- Evidence-Based Recommendations: Eat fresh or as part of a fruit salad.

5. Grapes
- Serving Size: 1 cup (151g)
- Phosphorus: 20 mg
- Calories: 104 kcal
- Nutritional Information: 1g protein, 27g carbohydrates, 0.2g fat, 288 mg potassium
- Medical Endorsement: Grapes are low in phosphorus and high in hydration.
- Evidence-Based Recommendations: Suitable as a snack or in fruit salads.

6. Strawberries
- Serving Size: 1 cup (152g)
- Phosphorus: 22 mg
- Calories: 49 kcal
- Nutritional Information: 1g protein, 12g carbohydrates, 0.5g fat, 220 mg potassium
- Medical Endorsement: Strawberries are low in phosphorus and high in vitamin C.
- Evidence-Based Recommendations: Enjoy fresh or in smoothies and salads.

7. Blueberries
- Serving Size: 1/2 cup (74g)
- Phosphorus: 10 mg
- Calories: 42 kcal

- Nutritional Information: 0.5g protein, 11g carbohydrates, 0.2g fat, 77 mg potassium
- Medical Endorsement: Blueberries are low in phosphorus and high in antioxidants.
- Evidence-Based Recommendations: Add to yogurt, cereals, or eat as a snack.

8. Raspberries
- Serving Size: 1 cup (123g)
- Phosphorus: 35 mg
- Calories: 65 kcal
- Nutritional Information: 1.5g protein, 15g carbohydrates, 0.8g fat, 186 mg potassium
- Medical Endorsement: Raspberries are low in phosphorus and rich in fiber.
- Evidence-Based Recommendations: Use in smoothies, desserts, or as a snack.

9. Watermelon
- Serving Size: 1 cup (152g)
- Phosphorus: 11 mg
- Calories: 46 kcal
- Nutritional Information: 1g protein, 12g carbohydrates, 0.2g fat, 170 mg potassium

- Medical Endorsement: Watermelon is low in phosphorus and helps with hydration.
- Evidence-Based Recommendations: Ideal for refreshing snacks or in fruit salads.

10. Cantaloupe
- Serving Size: 1 cup (160g)
- Phosphorus: 16 mg
- Calories: 53 kcal
- Nutritional Information: 1g protein, 14g carbohydrates, 0.3g fat, 417 mg potassium
- Medical Endorsement: Cantaloupe is low in phosphorus and provides vitamin A.
- Evidence-Based Recommendations: Enjoy fresh or in fruit salads.

11. Kiwi
- Serving Size: 1 medium kiwi (76g)
- Phosphorus: 24 mg
- Calories: 42 kcal
- Nutritional Information: 1g protein, 10g carbohydrates, 0.4g fat, 215 mg potassium
- Medical Endorsement: Kiwi is low in phosphorus and rich in vitamin C.
- Evidence-Based Recommendations: Eat fresh or add to fruit salads.

12. Tangerines
   - Serving Size: 1 medium tangerine (88g)
   - Phosphorus: 16 mg
   - Calories: 47 kcal
   - Nutritional Information: 0.6g protein, 12g carbohydrates, 0.2g fat, 130 mg potassium
   - Medical Endorsement: Tangerines are low in phosphorus and provide vitamin C.
   - Evidence-Based Recommendations: Enjoy as a snack or in fruit salads.

13. Apricots
   - Serving Size: 2 medium apricots (74g)
   - Phosphorus: 15 mg
   - Calories: 34 kcal
   - Nutritional Information: 0.5g protein, 9g carbohydrates, 0.2g fat, 130 mg potassium
   - Medical Endorsement: Apricots are low in phosphorus and high in vitamin A.
   - Evidence-Based Recommendations: Eat fresh or dried without added sugars.

14. Pineapple
   - Serving Size: 1 cup (165g)
   - Phosphorus: 13 mg
   - Calories: 82 kcal

- Nutritional Information: 0.5g protein, 22g carbohydrates, 0.2g fat, 180 mg potassium
- Medical Endorsement: Pineapple is low in phosphorus and high in vitamin C.
- Evidence-Based Recommendations: Enjoy fresh or in fruit salads and smoothies.

15. Coconut (Fresh)
   - Serving Size: 1/2 cup (46g)
   - Phosphorus: 13 mg
   - Calories: 140 kcal
   - Nutritional Information: 1.3g protein, 6g carbohydrates, 13g fat, 150 mg potassium
   - Medical Endorsement: Fresh coconut is low in phosphorus and provides healthy fats.
   - Evidence-Based Recommendations: Use in cooking or as a snack. Be mindful of portion sizes due to higher fat content.

Vegetables

1. Cucumber
   - Serving Size: 1 cup (104g)
   - Phosphorus: 24 mg
   - Calories: 16 kcal
   - Nutritional Information: 0.7g protein, 4g carbohydrates, 0.1g fat, 147 mg potassium
   - Medical Endorsement: Cucumber is low in phosphorus and very hydrating.
   - Evidence-Based Recommendations: Ideal for salads, snacks, or as a garnish.

2. Lettuce (Iceberg)
   - Serving Size: 1 cup (72g)
   - Phosphorus: 12 mg
   - Calories: 10 kcal
   - Nutritional Information: 0.5g protein, 2g carbohydrates, 0.1g fat, 116 mg potassium
   - Medical Endorsement: Iceberg lettuce is low in phosphorus and provides hydration.
   - Evidence-Based Recommendations: Use in salads, sandwiches, or wraps.

3. Zucchini
- Serving Size: 1 cup (124g)
- Phosphorus: 29 mg
- Calories: 19 kcal
- Nutritional Information: 1g protein, 4g carbohydrates, 0.3g fat, 295 mg potassium
- Medical Endorsement: Zucchini is low in phosphorus and versatile in cooking.
- Evidence-Based Recommendations: Suitable for grilling, sautéing, or adding to soups.

4. Bell Peppers (Red)
- Serving Size: 1 cup (92g)
- Phosphorus: 21 mg
- Calories: 31 kcal
- Nutritional Information: 1g protein, 7g carbohydrates, 0.3g fat, 200 mg potassium
- Medical Endorsement: Red bell peppers are low in phosphorus and rich in vitamin C.
- Evidence-Based Recommendations: Use in salads, stir-fries, or as a crunchy snack.

5. Cauliflower
- Serving Size: 1 cup (107g)
- Phosphorus: 33 mg
- Calories: 25 kcal

- Nutritional Information: 2g protein, 5g carbohydrates, 0.1g fat, 320 mg potassium
- Medical Endorsement: Cauliflower is low in phosphorus and can be used as a rice or mash substitute.
- Evidence-Based Recommendations: Roast, steam, or use in soups and casseroles.

6. Green Beans

- Serving Size: 1 cup (125g)
- Phosphorus: 30 mg
- Calories: 34 kcal
- Nutritional Information: 2g protein, 8g carbohydrates, 0.2g fat, 210 mg potassium
- Medical Endorsement: Green beans are low in phosphorus and a good source of fiber.
- Evidence-Based Recommendations: Steam, sauté, or use in salads and side dishes.

7. Radishes

- Serving Size: 1 cup (116g)
- Phosphorus: 20 mg
- Calories: 18 kcal
- Nutritional Information: 1g protein, 4g carbohydrates, 0.1g fat, 270 mg potassium

- Medical Endorsement: Radishes are low in phosphorus and provide a peppery flavor.
- Evidence-Based Recommendations: Eat raw in salads or as a crunchy snack.

8. Celery

- Serving Size: 1 cup (101g)
- Phosphorus: 27 mg
- Calories: 16 kcal
- Nutritional Information: 0.7g protein, 3g carbohydrates, 0.2g fat, 260 mg potassium
- Medical Endorsement: Celery is low in phosphorus and great for hydration.
- Evidence-Based Recommendations: Use in salads, soups, or as a snack with low-phosphorus dips.

9. Broccoli (Raw)

- Serving Size: 1 cup (91g)
- Phosphorus: 66 mg
- Calories: 31 kcal
- Nutritional Information: 3g protein, 6g carbohydrates, 0.4g fat, 288 mg potassium
- Medical Endorsement: Broccoli is slightly higher in phosphorus but still suitable in moderate amounts.

- Evidence-Based Recommendations: Steam or stir-fry as part of a balanced meal.

10. Spinach (Baby)
- Serving Size: 1 cup (30g)
- Phosphorus: 29 mg
- Calories: 7 kcal
- Nutritional Information: 1g protein, 1g carbohydrates, 0g fat, 167 mg potassium
- Medical Endorsement: Baby spinach is low in phosphorus but can be higher in potassium.
- Evidence-Based Recommendations: Use in salads or lightly cooked in dishes.

11. Asparagus
- Serving Size: 1 cup (134g)
- Phosphorus: 41 mg
- Calories: 27 kcal
- Nutritional Information: 3g protein, 5g carbohydrates, 0.2g fat, 270 mg potassium
- Medical Endorsement: Asparagus is low in phosphorus and provides antioxidants.
- Evidence-Based Recommendations: Grill, steam, or add to stir-fries and salads.

12. Mushrooms (White)
  - Serving Size: 1 cup (72g)
  - Phosphorus: 14 mg
  - Calories: 15 kcal
  - Nutritional Information: 2g protein, 3g carbohydrates, 0.2g fat, 223 mg potassium
  - Medical Endorsement: White mushrooms are low in phosphorus and versatile in cooking.
  - Evidence-Based Recommendations: Use in salads, soups, or sautéed as a side dish.

13. Squash (Butternut)
  - Serving Size: 1 cup (205g)
  - Phosphorus: 37 mg
  - Calories: 82 kcal
  - Nutritional Information: 1g protein, 22g carbohydrates, 0.2g fat, 582 mg potassium
  - Medical Endorsement: Butternut squash is low in phosphorus and high in vitamins.
  - Evidence-Based Recommendations: Roast, bake, or use in soups and stews.

14. Beets
  - Serving Size: 1 cup (136g)
  - Phosphorus: 40 mg
  - Calories: 59 kcal

- Nutritional Information: 2g protein, 13g carbohydrates, 0.2g fat, 305 mg potassium
- Medical Endorsement: Beets are moderate in phosphorus but rich in nutrients.
- Evidence-Based Recommendations: Roast, steam, or use in salads.

15. Pumpkin
- Serving Size: 1 cup (245g)
- Phosphorus: 56 mg
- Calories: 49 kcal
- Nutritional Information: 2g protein, 12g carbohydrates, 0.2g fat, 505 mg potassium
- Medical Endorsement: Pumpkin is low in phosphorus and provides fiber.
- Evidence-Based Recommendations: Use in soups, pies, or roasted as a side dish.

1. White Rice
   - Serving Size: 1 cup cooked (158g)
   - Phosphorus: 68 mg
   - Calories: 205 kcal
   - Nutritional Information: 4g protein, 45g carbohydrates, 0.4g fat, 26 mg potassium
   - Medical Endorsement: White rice is low in phosphorus compared to whole grains and is easy to digest.
   - Evidence-Based Recommendations: Ideal as a staple or side dish. Choose non-enriched varieties.

2. Cream of Rice Cereal
   - Serving Size: 1 cup cooked (240g)
   - Phosphorus: 18 mg
   - Calories: 100 kcal
   - Nutritional Information: 2g protein, 22g carbohydrates, 0.5g fat, 40 mg potassium
   - Medical Endorsement: Cream of rice is low in phosphorus and can be fortified with vitamins.
   - Evidence-Based Recommendations: Suitable for breakfast or as a base for other dishes.

3. White Pasta
* Serving Size: 1 cup cooked (140g)
* Phosphorus: 60 mg
* Calories: 220 kcal
* Nutritional Information: 8g protein, 43g carbohydrates, 1g fat, 53 mg potassium
* Medical Endorsement: White pasta is lower in phosphorus than whole-grain options.
* Evidence-Based Recommendations: Use in pasta dishes or salads. Avoid adding high-phosphorus sauces.

4. Polenta
* Serving Size: 1 cup cooked (240g)
* Phosphorus: 43 mg
* Calories: 130 kcal
* Nutritional Information: 3g protein, 28g carbohydrates, 0.6g fat, 140 mg potassium
* Medical Endorsement: Polenta is low in phosphorus and can be a versatile base for meals.
* Evidence-Based Recommendations: Serve as a side dish or base for sauces.

5. Cornmeal
* Serving Size: 1 cup cooked (160g)
* Phosphorus: 37 mg
* Calories: 120 kcal

- Nutritional Information: 3g protein, 29g carbohydrates, 0.5g fat, 228 mg potassium
- Medical Endorsement: Cornmeal is low in phosphorus and useful for baking or side dishes.
- Evidence-Based Recommendations: Use in cornbread, polenta, or as a coating for meats.

6. Oats (Instant)

- Serving Size: 1 cup cooked (234g)
- Phosphorus: 128 mg
- Calories: 150 kcal
- Nutritional Information: 6g protein, 27g carbohydrates, 2.5g fat, 160 mg potassium
- Medical Endorsement: Instant oats have higher phosphorus content; opt for small portions.
- Evidence-Based Recommendations: Suitable for breakfast; choose plain varieties without added phosphorus.

7. Quinoa (Cooked)

- Serving Size: 1 cup cooked (185g)
- Phosphorus: 280 mg
- Calories: 222 kcal
- Nutritional Information: 8g protein, 39g carbohydrates, 3.5g fat, 318 mg potassium

- Medical Endorsement: Quinoa is higher in phosphorus; moderate consumption is advised.
- Evidence-Based Recommendations: Use in moderation and consult with a dietitian for proper portioning.

8. Buckwheat (Cooked)

- Serving Size: 1 cup cooked (168g)
- Phosphorus: 86 mg
- Calories: 155 kcal
- Nutritional Information: 6g protein, 33g carbohydrates, 1g fat, 124 mg potassium
- Medical Endorsement: Buckwheat is lower in phosphorus and high in nutrients.
- Evidence-Based Recommendations: Use as a grain alternative or in salads.

9. Barley (Pearled, Cooked)

- Serving Size: 1 cup cooked (157g)
- Phosphorus: 76 mg
- Calories: 193 kcal
- Nutritional Information: 3.5g protein, 44g carbohydrates, 0.5g fat, 193 mg potassium
- Medical Endorsement: Pearled barley is lower in phosphorus and good for soups or stews.

- Evidence-Based Recommendations: Use in soups, salads, or as a side dish.

10. Farro (Cooked)
    - Serving Size: 1 cup cooked (140g)
    - Phosphorus: 110 mg
    - Calories: 170 kcal
    - Nutritional Information: 7g protein, 34g carbohydrates, 1g fat, 242 mg potassium
    - Medical Endorsement: Farro has moderate phosphorus content; consume in moderation.
    - Evidence-Based Recommendations: Ideal for salads or as a grain side dish.

11. Rice Cakes
    - Serving Size: 1 rice cake (9g)
    - Phosphorus: 10 mg
    - Calories: 35 kcal
    - Nutritional Information: 0.5g protein, 7g carbohydrates, 0g fat, 0 mg potassium
    - Medical Endorsement: Rice cakes are low in phosphorus and can be a snack option.
    - Evidence-Based Recommendations: Use as a snack or light meal base.

12. Polenta (Instant)
  - Serving Size: 1 cup cooked (240g)
  - Phosphorus: 43 mg
  - Calories: 130 kcal
  - Nutritional Information: 3g protein, 28g carbohydrates, 0.6g fat, 140 mg potassium
  - Medical Endorsement: Instant polenta is low in phosphorus and easy to prepare.
  - Evidence-Based Recommendations: Use as a base for vegetables or light meals.

13. Rice Noodles
  - Serving Size: 1 cup cooked (160g)
  - Phosphorus: 33 mg
  - Calories: 192 kcal
  - Nutritional Information: 2g protein, 43g carbohydrates, 1g fat, 30 mg potassium
  - Medical Endorsement: Rice noodles are low in phosphorus and suitable for various dishes.
  - Evidence-Based Recommendations: Use in soups, stir-fries, or as a pasta alternative.

14. Puffed Rice
  - Serving Size: 1 cup (30g)
  - Phosphorus: 15 mg
  - Calories: 100 kcal

- Nutritional Information: 2g protein, 22g carbohydrates, 0g fat, 0 mg potassium
- Medical Endorsement: Puffed rice is low in phosphorus and can be used as a snack or cereal base.
- Evidence-Based Recommendations: Suitable for breakfast or as a light snack.

15. Couscous (Plain)
  - Serving Size: 1 cup cooked (157g)
  - Phosphorus: 64 mg
  - Calories: 176 kcal
  - Nutritional Information: 6g protein, 36g carbohydrates, 0.3g fat, 176 mg potassium
  - Medical Endorsement: Couscous is low in phosphorus and versatile in dishes.
  - Evidence-Based Recommendations: Use in salads, as a side dish, or with low-phosphorus proteins.

1. Apple Slices with Almond Butter
   - Serving Size: 1 medium apple with 1 tablespoon almond butter
   - Phosphorus: 29 mg (apple) + 50 mg (almond butter) = 79 mg
   - Calories: 95 kcal (apple) + 98 kcal (almond butter) = 193 kcal
   - Nutritional Information: 1g protein (apple), 3g protein (almond butter), 25g carbohydrates (apple), 4g carbohydrates (almond butter), 0.3g fat (apple), 9g fat (almond butter), 160 mg potassium (apple), 93 mg potassium (almond butter)
   - Medical Endorsement: Apples are low in phosphorus; almond butter should be used in moderation due to higher phosphorus.
   - Evidence-Based Recommendations: A balanced snack with fruit and a small amount of nut butter. Choose natural, unsweetened almond butter.

2. Rice Cakes with Cucumber Slices
   - Serving Size: 2 rice cakes with 1/2 cup cucumber slices
   - Phosphorus: 20 mg (rice cakes) + 12 mg (cucumber) = 32 mg

- Calories: 70 kcal (rice cakes) + 8 kcal (cucumber) = 78 kcal
- Nutritional Information: 1g protein (rice cakes), 0.5g protein (cucumber), 15g carbohydrates (rice cakes), 2g carbohydrates (cucumber), 0g fat (rice cakes), 0.1g fat (cucumber), 0 mg potassium (rice cakes), 116 mg potassium (cucumber)
- Medical Endorsement: Both rice cakes and cucumbers are low in phosphorus and provide a light, refreshing snack.
- Evidence-Based Recommendations: Ideal for a low-phosphorus, hydrating snack.

3. Puffed Rice with Fresh Berries
- Serving Size: 1 cup puffed rice with 1/2 cup fresh strawberries
- Phosphorus: 15 mg (puffed rice) + 20 mg (strawberries) = 35 mg
- Calories: 100 kcal (puffed rice) + 25 kcal (strawberries) = 125 kcal
- Nutritional Information: 2g protein (puffed rice), 0.5g protein (strawberries), 22g carbohydrates (puffed rice), 6g carbohydrates (strawberries), 0g fat (puffed rice), 0.2g fat (strawberries), 0 mg potassium (puffed rice), 160 mg potassium (strawberries)

- Medical Endorsement: Puffed rice and strawberries are both low in phosphorus, making for a light, sweet snack.
- Evidence-Based Recommendations: Suitable for a low-phosphorus, fruit-based snack.

4. Carrot Sticks with Hummus

- Serving Size: 1 cup carrot sticks with 2 tablespoons hummus
- Phosphorus: 25 mg (carrots) + 40 mg (hummus) = 65 mg
- Calories: 50 kcal (carrots) + 70 kcal (hummus) = 120 kcal
- Nutritional Information: 1g protein (carrots), 2g protein (hummus), 12g carbohydrates (carrots), 6g carbohydrates (hummus), 0g fat (carrots), 5g fat (hummus), 320 mg potassium (carrots), 90 mg potassium (hummus)
- Medical Endorsement: Carrots are low in phosphorus; hummus should be used sparingly due to its phosphorus content.
- Evidence-Based Recommendations: Ideal as a crunchy, nutritious snack.

5. Plain Greek Yogurt (Low Phosphorus)
   - Serving Size: 1/2 cup plain Greek yogurt
   - Phosphorus: 90 mg
   - Calories: 80 kcal
   - Nutritional Information: 10g protein, 6g carbohydrates, 2g fat, 180 mg potassium
   - Medical Endorsement: Opt for low-phosphorus Greek yogurt and consume in moderation.
   - Evidence-Based Recommendations: Suitable for a protein-rich snack. Avoid flavored varieties with added phosphorus.

6. Rice Pudding (Homemade)
   - Serving Size: 1/2 cup homemade rice pudding
   - Phosphorus: 55 mg
   - Calories: 150 kcal
   - Nutritional Information: 3g protein, 22g carbohydrates, 5g fat, 140 mg potassium
   - Medical Endorsement: Rice pudding made with low-phosphorus ingredients can be a comforting snack.
   - Evidence-Based Recommendations: Ideal for a sweet treat. Ensure low-phosphorus ingredients are used.

7. Cantaloupe Cubes
  - Serving Size: 1 cup cantaloupe cubes
  - Phosphorus: 17 mg
  - Calories: 53 kcal
  - Nutritional Information: 1g protein, 14g carbohydrates, 0g fat, 300 mg potassium
  - Medical Endorsement: Cantaloupe is low in phosphorus and high in water content.
  - Evidence-Based Recommendations: Excellent for hydration and a refreshing, low-phosphorus snack.

8. Celery Sticks with Cream Cheese
  - Serving Size: 3 celery sticks with 2 tablespoons cream cheese
  - Phosphorus: 27 mg (celery) + 40 mg (cream cheese) = 67 mg
  - Calories: 16 kcal (celery) + 100 kcal (cream cheese) = 116 kcal
  - Nutritional Information: 0.7g protein (celery), 2g protein (cream cheese), 3g carbohydrates (celery), 1g carbohydrates (cream cheese), 0.2g fat (celery), 10g fat (cream cheese), 260 mg potassium (celery), 60 mg potassium (cream cheese)
  - Medical Endorsement: Celery is low in phosphorus; cream cheese should be

used in small amounts due to its phosphorus content.
- Evidence-Based Recommendations: A crunchy snack with a creamy addition.

9. Homemade Apple Chips
- Serving Size: 1 ounce apple chips
- Phosphorus: 15 mg
- Calories: 60 kcal
- Nutritional Information: 0g protein, 16g carbohydrates, 0g fat, 70 mg potassium
- Medical Endorsement: Apple chips are low in phosphorus and provide a crunchy alternative to fresh fruit.
- Evidence-Based Recommendations: Make homemade apple chips to avoid added phosphorus.

10. Boiled White Potatoes
- Serving Size: 1 small boiled potato (150g)
- Phosphorus: 27 mg
- Calories: 130 kcal
- Nutritional Information: 3g protein, 30g carbohydrates, 0g fat, 620 mg potassium
- Medical Endorsement: White potatoes are low in phosphorus and high in potassium.

- Evidence-Based Recommendations: Eat plain or with low-phosphorus seasonings.

11. Popped Popcorn (Lightly Salted)
    - Serving Size: 1 cup popped popcorn
    - Phosphorus: 30 mg
    - Calories: 31 kcal
    - Nutritional Information: 1g protein, 6g carbohydrates, 0g fat, 10 mg potassium
    - Medical Endorsement: Popcorn is low in phosphorus; avoid added salt or butter.
    - Evidence-Based Recommendations: Ideal for a light, crunchy snack.

12. Pear Slices
    - Serving Size: 1 medium pear (178g)
    - Phosphorus: 22 mg
    - Calories: 102 kcal
    - Nutritional Information: 1g protein, 27g carbohydrates, 0g fat, 190 mg potassium
    - Medical Endorsement: Pears are low in phosphorus and hydrating.
    - Evidence-Based Recommendations: Fresh pear slices make a refreshing, low-phosphorus snack.

13. Grapes

- Serving Size: 1 cup grapes
- Phosphorus: 22 mg
- Calories: 104 kcal
- Nutritional Information: 1g protein, 27g carbohydrates, 0g fat, 288 mg potassium
- Medical Endorsement: Grapes are low in phosphorus and high in antioxidants.
- Evidence-Based Recommendations: Great as a fresh, sweet snack.

14. Peach Slices

- Serving Size: 1 medium peach (150g)
- Phosphorus: 24 mg
- Calories: 59 kcal
- Nutritional Information: 1g protein, 15g carbohydrates, 0g fat, 285 mg potassium
- Medical Endorsement: Peaches are low in phosphorus and hydrating.
- Evidence-Based Recommendations: Fresh peaches are ideal for a light, low-phosphorus snack.

15. Low-Fat Vanilla Yogurt

- Serving Size: 1/2 cup low-fat vanilla yogurt
- Phosphorus: 80 mg
- Calories: 75 kcal

- Nutritional Information: 4g protein, 12g carbohydrates, 0g fat, 100 mg potassium
- Medical Endorsement: Opt for low-fat varieties with low phosphorus content.
- Evidence-Based Recommendations: Suitable for a light, creamy snack. Avoid varieties with added phosphates.

Proteins

1. Egg Whites
   - Serving Size: 3 large egg whites (100g)
   - Phosphorus: 7 mg
   - Calories: 51 kcal
   - Nutritional Information: 11g protein, 0g carbohydrates, 0g fat, 163 mg potassium
   - Medical Endorsement: Egg whites are low in phosphorus and provide high-quality protein without additional phosphorus.
   - Evidence-Based Recommendations: Suitable for a low-phosphorus diet. Use in omelets or scrambled eggs.

2. Chicken Breast (Cooked)
   - Serving Size: 3 oz (85g)
   - Phosphorus: 170 mg
   - Calories: 140 kcal

- Nutritional Information: 26g protein, 0g carbohydrates, 3g fat, 300 mg potassium
- Medical Endorsement: Chicken breast is a good source of lean protein and relatively low in phosphorus.
- Evidence-Based Recommendations: Use as a main protein source, ensuring to avoid high-phosphorus seasonings.

3. Turkey Breast (Cooked)
- Serving Size: 3 oz (85g)
- Phosphorus: 150 mg
- Calories: 135 kcal
- Nutritional Information: 25g protein, 0g carbohydrates, 1g fat, 270 mg potassium
- Medical Endorsement: Turkey breast is low in phosphorus and a lean protein option.
- Evidence-Based Recommendations: Ideal for sandwiches or as a main dish.

4. Cod (Cooked)
- Serving Size: 3 oz (85g)
- Phosphorus: 140 mg
- Calories: 90 kcal
- Nutritional Information: 20g protein, 0g carbohydrates, 0.5g fat, 300 mg potassium

- Medical Endorsement: Cod is low in phosphorus and a good source of protein.
- Evidence-Based Recommendations: Suitable for baking or grilling.

5. Tuna (Canned in Water)
- Serving Size: 3 oz (85g)
- Phosphorus: 160 mg
- Calories: 100 kcal
- Nutritional Information: 22g protein, 0g carbohydrates, 0.5g fat, 200 mg potassium
- Medical Endorsement: Tuna is low in phosphorus, especially when packed in water.
- Evidence-Based Recommendations: Use in salads or sandwiches, but limit intake to avoid mercury accumulation.

6. Shrimp (Cooked)
- Serving Size: 3 oz (85g)
- Phosphorus: 225 mg
- Calories: 84 kcal
- Nutritional Information: 20g protein, 0g carbohydrates, 1g fat, 200 mg potassium
- Medical Endorsement: Shrimp is low in phosphorus but should be consumed in moderation.

- Evidence-Based Recommendations: Ideal for stir-fries or as a protein addition to salads.

7. Tofu (Firm)
  - Serving Size: 3 oz (85g)
  - Phosphorus: 80 mg
  - Calories: 70 kcal
  - Nutritional Information: 8g protein, 2g carbohydrates, 4g fat, 150 mg potassium
  - Medical Endorsement: Firm tofu is relatively low in phosphorus and a good plant-based protein option.
  - Evidence-Based Recommendations: Use in stir-fries or salads.

8. Greek Yogurt (Plain, Low-Fat)
  - Serving Size: 1/2 cup (125g)
  - Phosphorus: 90 mg
  - Calories: 75 kcal
  - Nutritional Information: 10g protein, 6g carbohydrates, 2g fat, 150 mg potassium
  - Medical Endorsement: Plain Greek yogurt is low in phosphorus and provides high-quality protein.
  - Evidence-Based Recommendations: Suitable for breakfast or snacks. Opt for plain varieties without added sugars.

9. Cottage Cheese (Low-Fat)
- Serving Size: 1/2 cup (113g)
- Phosphorus: 200 mg
- Calories: 90 kcal
- Nutritional Information: 12g protein, 4g carbohydrates, 1g fat, 200 mg potassium
- Medical Endorsement: Low-fat cottage cheese is a good protein source but should be consumed in moderation.
- Evidence-Based Recommendations: Use as a snack or in recipes. Opt for low-sodium versions.

10. Egg Substitute (Liquid)
- Serving Size: 1/4 cup (60g)
- Phosphorus: 50 mg
- Calories: 30 kcal
- Nutritional Information: 7g protein, 0g carbohydrates, 0g fat, 100 mg potassium
- Medical Endorsement: Egg substitutes are low in phosphorus and can replace whole eggs in recipes.
- Evidence-Based Recommendations: Use in cooking or baking as a lower-phosphorus alternative to whole eggs.

11. Chicken Sausage (Low-Sodium)
   - Serving Size: 1 sausage (85g)
   - Phosphorus: 150 mg
   - Calories: 160 kcal
   - Nutritional Information: 12g protein, 2g carbohydrates, 10g fat, 200 mg potassium
   - Medical Endorsement: Low-sodium chicken sausage provides a lower-phosphorus option compared to regular sausages.
   - Evidence-Based Recommendations: Use in moderation and ensure low-sodium varieties.

12. Lean Beef (Cooked)
   - Serving Size: 3 oz (85g)
   - Phosphorus: 215 mg
   - Calories: 180 kcal
   - Nutritional Information: 22g protein, 0g carbohydrates, 9g fat, 310 mg potassium
   - Medical Endorsement: Lean beef is relatively high in phosphorus; consume in moderation.
   - Evidence-Based Recommendations: Choose lean cuts and limit portion sizes to manage phosphorus intake.

13. Pork Tenderloin (Cooked)
- Serving Size: 3 oz (85g)
- Phosphorus: 175 mg
- Calories: 140 kcal
- Nutritional Information: 22g protein, 0g carbohydrates, 6g fat, 290 mg potassium
- Medical Endorsement: Pork tenderloin is a lower-phosphorus option compared to other cuts of pork.
- Evidence-Based Recommendations: Ideal as a main protein source, ensuring to avoid high-phosphorus seasonings.

14. Low-Phosphorus Protein Powder (Unflavored)
- Serving Size: 1 scoop (30g)
- Phosphorus: 80 mg
- Calories: 120 kcal
- Nutritional Information: 20g protein, 2g carbohydrates, 1g fat, 150 mg potassium
- Medical Endorsement: Low-phosphorus protein powder can be useful for meeting protein needs without excessive phosphorus.
- Evidence-Based Recommendations: Use as a supplement to meals or as a shake. Check for added phosphorus in the ingredients.

15. Fish (Tilapia, Cooked)
  - Serving Size: 3 oz (85g)
  - Phosphorus: 240 mg
  - Calories: 120 kcal
  - Nutritional Information: 21g protein, 0g carbohydrates, 2g fat, 300 mg potassium
  - Medical Endorsement: Tilapia is lower in phosphorus compared to other fish and provides lean protein.
  - Evidence-Based Recommendations: Ideal for grilling or baking. Limit high-phosphorus sauces.

Dairy Alternatives

1. Almond Milk (Unsweetened)
  - Serving Size: 1 cup (240 ml)
  - Phosphorus: 25 mg
  - Calories: 30 kcal
  - Nutritional Information: 1g protein, 1g carbohydrates, 2.5g fat, 160 mg potassium
  - Medical Endorsement: Unsweetened almond milk is low in phosphorus and can be a good substitute for dairy milk.
  - Evidence-Based Recommendations: Opt for fortified versions if additional calcium and vitamin D are needed.

2. Rice Milk (Unsweetened)
- Serving Size: 1 cup (240 ml)
- Phosphorus: 30 mg
- Calories: 50 kcal
- Nutritional Information: 1g protein, 10g carbohydrates, 1.5g fat, 160 mg potassium
- Medical Endorsement: Rice milk is low in phosphorus and provides a mild, sweet flavor.
- Evidence-Based Recommendations: Choose unsweetened varieties to avoid added sugars.

3. Coconut Milk (Unsweetened)
- Serving Size: 1 cup (240 ml)
- Phosphorus: 20 mg
- Calories: 45 kcal
- Nutritional Information: 0.5g protein, 1g carbohydrates, 4.5g fat, 250 mg potassium
- Medical Endorsement: Unsweetened coconut milk is low in phosphorus and can be used in cooking or as a beverage.
- Evidence-Based Recommendations: Ensure it is fortified with calcium and vitamin D if used as a milk replacement.

4. Cashew Milk (Unsweetened)
  - Serving Size: 1 cup (240 ml)
  - Phosphorus: 35 mg
  - Calories: 25 kcal
  - Nutritional Information: 1g protein, 1g carbohydrates, 2g fat, 160 mg potassium
  - Medical Endorsement: Cashew milk is low in phosphorus and provides a creamy texture.
  - Evidence-Based Recommendations: Choose unsweetened varieties to avoid added sugars.

5. Oat Milk (Unsweetened)
  - Serving Size: 1 cup (240 ml)
  - Phosphorus: 40 mg
  - Calories: 60 kcal
  - Nutritional Information: 2g protein, 15g carbohydrates, 2.5g fat, 350 mg potassium
  - Medical Endorsement: Oat milk is slightly higher in phosphorus but can be used in moderation.
  - Evidence-Based Recommendations: Opt for unsweetened varieties and monitor portion sizes.

6. Hemp Milk (Unsweetened)
  - Serving Size: 1 cup (240 ml)
  - Phosphorus: 35 mg
  - Calories: 60 kcal
  - Nutritional Information: 3g protein, 1g carbohydrates, 5g fat, 250 mg potassium
  - Medical Endorsement: Hemp milk is low in phosphorus and provides additional omega-3 fatty acids.
  - Evidence-Based Recommendations: Choose unsweetened versions and check for added nutrients like calcium.

7. Soy Milk (Unsweetened)
  - Serving Size: 1 cup (240 ml)
  - Phosphorus: 60 mg
  - Calories: 80 kcal
  - Nutritional Information: 7g protein, 4g carbohydrates, 4g fat, 300 mg potassium
  - Medical Endorsement: Soy milk has a moderate phosphorus content; opt for unsweetened versions to reduce additional phosphorus.
  - Evidence-Based Recommendations: Suitable for use in cooking and as a milk replacement.

8. Almond-Based Yogurt (Unsweetened)
- Serving Size: 1/2 cup (120g)
- Phosphorus: 50 mg
- Calories: 60 kcal
- Nutritional Information: 2g protein, 6g carbohydrates, 2g fat, 120 mg potassium
- Medical Endorsement: Almond-based yogurt is low in phosphorus and can be used as a snack or in recipes.
- Evidence-Based Recommendations: Choose unsweetened and fortified versions for added nutritional benefits.

9. Coconut-Based Yogurt (Unsweetened)
- Serving Size: 1/2 cup (120g)
- Phosphorus: 40 mg
- Calories: 90 kcal
- Nutritional Information: 1g protein, 6g carbohydrates, 8g fat, 150 mg potassium
- Medical Endorsement: Coconut-based yogurt is low in phosphorus and provides a rich, creamy texture.
- Evidence-Based Recommendations: Ideal for snacks or as a breakfast option. Ensure it is fortified with calcium.

10. Cashew-Based Yogurt (Unsweetened)
  - Serving Size: 1/2 cup (120g)
  - Phosphorus: 55 mg
  - Calories: 80 kcal
  - Nutritional Information: 2g protein, 7g carbohydrates, 4g fat, 130 mg potassium
  - Medical Endorsement: Cashew-based yogurt is low in phosphorus and provides a creamy alternative to dairy yogurt.
  - Evidence-Based Recommendations: Use as a snack or part of a meal.

11. Rice-Based Yogurt (Unsweetened)
  - Serving Size: 1/2 cup (120g)
  - Phosphorus: 60 mg
  - Calories: 70 kcal
  - Nutritional Information: 2g protein, 10g carbohydrates, 2g fat, 140 mg potassium
  - Medical Endorsement: Rice-based yogurt is relatively low in phosphorus and can be a good dairy alternative.
  - Evidence-Based Recommendations: Opt for unsweetened versions and check for added calcium and vitamins.

12. Soy-Based Cream Cheese (Low-Phosphorus)
- Serving Size: 2 tablespoons (30g)
- Phosphorus: 60 mg
- Calories: 90 kcal
- Nutritional Information: 3g protein, 2g carbohydrates, 8g fat, 150 mg potassium
- Medical Endorsement: Soy-based cream cheese is lower in phosphorus compared to dairy cream cheese.
- Evidence-Based Recommendations: Use as a spread or in recipes. Ensure it is low-sodium.

13. Almond-Based Creamer (Unsweetened)
- Serving Size: 2 tablespoons (30 ml)
- Phosphorus: 10 mg
- Calories: 15 kcal
- Nutritional Information: 0g protein, 1g carbohydrates, 1.5g fat, 60 mg potassium
- Medical Endorsement: Almond-based creamer is low in phosphorus and can be used to enhance coffee or tea.
- Evidence-Based Recommendations: Choose unsweetened and check for added nutrients like calcium.

14. Coconut-Based Creamer (Unsweetened)
  - Serving Size: 2 tablespoons (30 ml)
  - Phosphorus: 15 mg
  - Calories: 25 kcal
  - Nutritional Information: 0g protein, 2g carbohydrates, 2g fat, 80 mg potassium
  - Medical Endorsement: Coconut-based creamer is low in phosphorus and adds a subtle flavor to beverages.
  - Evidence-Based Recommendations: Use in moderation and check for added vitamins.

15. Hemp-Based Creamer (Unsweetened)
  - Serving Size: 2 tablespoons (30 ml)
  - Phosphorus: 20 mg
  - Calories: 25 kcal
  - Nutritional Information: 0g protein, 2g carbohydrates, 2g fat, 90 mg potassium
  - Medical Endorsement: Hemp-based creamer is low in phosphorus and can be used to add creaminess to drinks.
  - Evidence-Based Recommendations: Opt for unsweetened varieties and check for additional nutrients.

Herbs and spices

1. Basil (Fresh)
   - Serving Size: 1 tablespoon (2g)
   - Phosphorus: 7 mg
   - Calories: 1 kcal
   - Nutritional Information: 0g protein, 0g carbohydrates, 0g fat, 5 mg potassium
   - Medical Endorsement: Fresh basil is low in phosphorus and adds flavor to dishes without adding excess sodium.
   - Evidence-Based Recommendations: Use in salads, pasta sauces, or as a garnish.

2. Cilantro (Fresh)
   - Serving Size: 1 tablespoon (2g)
   - Phosphorus: 8 mg
   - Calories: 1 kcal
   - Nutritional Information: 0g protein, 0g carbohydrates, 0g fat, 10 mg potassium
   - Medical Endorsement: Cilantro is low in phosphorus and can enhance the flavor of a variety of dishes.
   - Evidence-Based Recommendations: Ideal for use in salsas, salads, or as a garnish.

3. Chives (Fresh)
- Serving Size: 1 tablespoon (2g)
- Phosphorus: 6 mg
- Calories: 1 kcal
- Nutritional Information: 0g protein, 0g carbohydrates, 0g fat, 6 mg potassium
- Medical Endorsement: Chives are low in phosphorus and provide a mild onion flavor.
- Evidence-Based Recommendations: Use as a garnish for soups, salads, and dishes.

4. Dill (Fresh)
- Serving Size: 1 tablespoon (2g)
- Phosphorus: 7 mg
- Calories: 1 kcal
- Nutritional Information: 0g protein, 0g carbohydrates, 0g fat, 9 mg potassium
- Medical Endorsement: Dill is low in phosphorus and adds a fresh, herbal flavor to foods.
- Evidence-Based Recommendations: Use in fish dishes, salads, or as a garnish.

5. Mint (Fresh)
- Serving Size: 1 tablespoon (2g)
- Phosphorus: 8 mg
- Calories: 1 kcal

- Nutritional Information: 0g protein, 0g carbohydrates, 0g fat, 7 mg potassium
- Medical Endorsement: Fresh mint is low in phosphorus and adds a refreshing flavor.
- Evidence-Based Recommendations: Use in teas, salads, or as a garnish.

6. Oregano (Dried)
- Serving Size: 1 teaspoon (1g)
- Phosphorus: 10 mg
- Calories: 3 kcal
- Nutritional Information: 0.1g protein, 0.6g carbohydrates, 0.1g fat, 10 mg potassium
- Medical Endorsement: Dried oregano is low in phosphorus and provides a robust flavor to dishes.
- Evidence-Based Recommendations: Ideal for use in Italian dishes, sauces, and soups.

7. Rosemary (Fresh)
- Serving Size: 1 tablespoon (2g)
- Phosphorus: 10 mg
- Calories: 3 kcal
- Nutritional Information: 0.1g protein, 0.6g carbohydrates, 0.1g fat, 10 mg potassium

- Medical Endorsement: Fresh rosemary is low in phosphorus and imparts a strong, aromatic flavor.
- Evidence-Based Recommendations: Use in roasted dishes, marinades, and as a flavor enhancer.

8. Thyme (Fresh)
- Serving Size: 1 tablespoon (2g)
- Phosphorus: 8 mg
- Calories: 1 kcal
- Nutritional Information: 0g protein, 0g carbohydrates, 0g fat, 6 mg potassium
- Medical Endorsement: Thyme is low in phosphorus and adds a subtle, earthy flavor.
- Evidence-Based Recommendations: Use in soups, stews, and roasted vegetables.

9. Paprika (Ground)
- Serving Size: 1 teaspoon (2g)
- Phosphorus: 8 mg
- Calories: 6 kcal
- Nutritional Information: 0.3g protein, 1.2g carbohydrates, 0.3g fat, 50 mg potassium
- Medical Endorsement: Paprika is low in phosphorus and adds color and mild heat to dishes.

- Evidence-Based Recommendations: Use in seasoning blends, soups, and stews.

10. Turmeric (Ground)
- Serving Size: 1 teaspoon (2g)
- Phosphorus: 10 mg
- Calories: 6 kcal
- Nutritional Information: 0.2g protein, 1.4g carbohydrates, 0.2g fat, 50 mg potassium
- Medical Endorsement: Turmeric is low in phosphorus and provides a vibrant color and earthy flavor.
- Evidence-Based Recommendations: Use in curries, rice dishes, and marinades.

11. Ginger (Ground)
- Serving Size: 1 teaspoon (2g)
- Phosphorus: 7 mg
- Calories: 6 kcal
- Nutritional Information: 0.2g protein, 1.2g carbohydrates, 0.1g fat, 20 mg potassium
- Medical Endorsement: Ground ginger is low in phosphorus and adds a spicy, warming flavor.
- Evidence-Based Recommendations: Use in baked goods, teas, and stir-fries.

12. Garlic Powder (Low-Sodium)

- Serving Size: 1 teaspoon (2g)
- Phosphorus: 6 mg
- Calories: 8 kcal
- Nutritional Information: 0.3g protein, 2g carbohydrates, 0g fat, 15 mg potassium
- Medical Endorsement: Garlic powder is low in phosphorus and can enhance the flavor of dishes without added sodium.
- Evidence-Based Recommendations: Use in seasoning blends and for adding depth of flavor to various dishes.

13. Cumin (Ground)

- Serving Size: 1 teaspoon (2g)
- Phosphorus: 14 mg
- Calories: 8 kcal
- Nutritional Information: 0.4g protein, 1.3g carbohydrates, 0.4g fat, 50 mg potassium
- Medical Endorsement: Cumin is relatively low in phosphorus and adds a warm, earthy flavor.
- Evidence-Based Recommendations: Ideal for use in spice blends, stews, and Mexican dishes.

14. Fennel Seeds
- Serving Size: 1 teaspoon (2g)
- Phosphorus: 13 mg
- Calories: 8 kcal
- Nutritional Information: 0.4g protein, 1.4g carbohydrates, 0.4g fat, 35 mg potassium
- Medical Endorsement: Fennel seeds are low in phosphorus and can provide a sweet, anise-like flavor.
- Evidence-Based Recommendations: Use in seasoning blends and as a digestive aid.

15. Bay Leaves (Dried)
- Serving Size: 1 leaf (0.5g)
- Phosphorus: 2 mg
- Calories: 1 kcal
- Nutritional Information: 0.1g protein, 0.3g carbohydrates, 0.1g fat, 5 mg potassium
- Medical Endorsement: Bay leaves are very low in phosphorus and add depth of flavor to slow-cooked dishes.
- Evidence-Based Recommendations: Use in soups, stews, and braises. Remove before serving.

Fruits

1. Apple
- Serving Size: 1 medium apple (182g)
- Potassium: 195 mg
- Calories: 95 kcal
- Nutritional Information: 0.5g protein, 25g carbohydrates, 0.3g fat, 4g fiber
- Medical Endorsement: Apples are low in potassium and provide fiber, which can help with digestion.
- Evidence-Based Recommendations: Ideal for snacking, baking, or adding to salads.

2. Blueberries
- Serving Size: 1/2 cup (74g)
- Potassium: 65 mg
- Calories: 42 kcal
- Nutritional Information: 0.5g protein, 11g carbohydrates, 0.2g fat, 1.8g fiber
- Medical Endorsement: Blueberries are low in potassium and high in antioxidants, which are beneficial for overall health.
- Evidence-Based Recommendations: Great for adding to cereals, yogurt, or smoothies.

3. Cranberries
   - Serving Size: 1/2 cup (50g)
   - Potassium: 44 mg
   - Calories: 25 kcal
   - Nutritional Information: 0.1g protein, 6.6g carbohydrates, 0.1g fat, 2g fiber
   - Medical Endorsement: Cranberries are very low in potassium and can help prevent urinary tract infections.
   - Evidence-Based Recommendations: Can be consumed fresh, dried, or as juice (in moderation).

4. Pineapple
   - Serving Size: 1/2 cup (82g)
   - Potassium: 88 mg
   - Calories: 41 kcal
   - Nutritional Information: 0.5g protein, 11g carbohydrates, 0.1g fat, 1.2g fiber
   - Medical Endorsement: Pineapple is low in potassium and provides vitamin C, which supports immune function.
   - Evidence-Based Recommendations: Enjoy fresh or in fruit salads.

5. Strawberries
   - Serving Size: 1/2 cup (76g)
   - Potassium: 120 mg
   - Calories: 27 kcal
   - Nutritional Information: 0.6g protein, 6.5g carbohydrates, 0.2g fat, 2g fiber

- Medical Endorsement: Strawberries are low in potassium and rich in antioxidants.
- Evidence-Based Recommendations: Can be eaten fresh, in smoothies, or as a topping for cereals.

6. Raspberries
- Serving Size: 1/2 cup (62g)
- Potassium: 93 mg
- Calories: 32 kcal
- Nutritional Information: 0.7g protein, 7g carbohydrates, 0.3g fat, 4g fiber
- Medical Endorsement: Raspberries are low in potassium and high in fiber, which can aid digestion.
- Evidence-Based Recommendations: Use in smoothies, desserts, or as a snack.

7. Peach
- Serving Size: 1 small peach (130g)
- Potassium: 190 mg
- Calories: 51 kcal
- Nutritional Information: 1g protein, 13g carbohydrates, 0.3g fat, 2g fiber
- Medical Endorsement: Peaches are low in potassium and provide vitamins A and C.

- Evidence-Based Recommendations: Enjoy fresh, canned (in water or juice), or as part of a dessert.

8. Grapes
- Serving Size: 1/2 cup (75g)
- Potassium: 144 mg
- Calories: 52 kcal
- Nutritional Information: 0.5g protein, 14g carbohydrates, 0.2g fat, 0.7g fiber
- Medical Endorsement: Grapes are low in potassium and are a good source of antioxidants.
- Evidence-Based Recommendations: Ideal as a snack, in salads, or as a dessert.

9. Watermelon
- Serving Size: 1 cup, diced (152g)
- Potassium: 170 mg
- Calories: 46 kcal
- Nutritional Information: 0.9g protein, 11.6g carbohydrates, 0.2g fat, 0.6g fiber
- Medical Endorsement: Watermelon is low in potassium and has high water content, making it hydrating.
- Evidence-Based Recommendations: Enjoy fresh or in fruit salads during hot weather.

10. Applesauce (Unsweetened)
   - Serving Size: 1/2 cup (122g)
   - Potassium: 90 mg
   - Calories: 50 kcal
   - Nutritional Information: 0.1g protein, 13g carbohydrates, 0g fat, 1.5g fiber
   - Medical Endorsement: Applesauce is low in potassium and easy to digest.
   - Evidence-Based Recommendations: Great as a snack or dessert option.

11. Plums
   - Serving Size: 1 small plum (66g)
   - Potassium: 104 mg
   - Calories: 30 kcal
   - Nutritional Information: 0.5g protein, 7.5g carbohydrates, 0.2g fat, 0.9g fiber
   - Medical Endorsement: Plums are low in potassium and rich in vitamins and antioxidants.
   - Evidence-Based Recommendations: Enjoy fresh or as a snack.

12. Tangerines
   - Serving Size: 1 medium tangerine (109g)
   - Potassium: 132 mg
   - Calories: 50 kcal
   - Nutritional Information: 0.8g protein, 13g carbohydrates, 0.3g fat, 1.7g fiber

- Medical Endorsement: Tangerines are low in potassium and provide a good source of vitamin C.
- Evidence-Based Recommendations: Ideal for snacking or adding to salads.

13. Cranberry Juice
   - Serving Size: 1/2 cup (125 ml)
   - Potassium: 22 mg
   - Calories: 60 kcal
   - Nutritional Information: 0g protein, 16g carbohydrates, 0g fat, 0g fiber
   - Medical Endorsement: Cranberry juice is very low in potassium and can help prevent urinary tract infections.
   - Evidence-Based Recommendations: Consume in moderation due to sugar content.

14. Blackberries
   - Serving Size: 1/2 cup (72g)
   - Potassium: 117 mg
   - Calories: 31 kcal
   - Nutritional Information: 1g protein, 7g carbohydrates, 0.3g fat, 3.8g fiber
   - Medical Endorsement: Blackberries are low in potassium and high in fiber and antioxidants.
   - Evidence-Based Recommendations: Ideal for snacking, in smoothies, or as a dessert topping.

15. Canned Pears (in Juice, Drained)
  - Serving Size: 1/2 cup (120g)
  - Potassium: 95 mg
  - Calories: 60 kcal
  - Nutritional Information: 0g protein, 16g carbohydrates, 0g fat, 2g fiber
  - Medical Endorsement: Canned pears are low in potassium and easy to digest.
  - Evidence-Based Recommendations: Can be used in salads, desserts, or as a snack.

Dairy Alternatives

1. Almond Milk (Unsweetened)
  - Serving Size: 1 cup (240ml)
  - Potassium: 180 mg
  - Calories: 30 kcal
  - Nutritional Information: 1g protein, 1g carbohydrates, 2.5g fat, 0g fiber
  - Medical Endorsement: Almond milk is a low-potassium alternative to cow's milk and is often fortified with calcium and vitamin D.
  - Evidence-Based Recommendations: Use in cereals, smoothies, or as a milk substitute in recipes.

2. Rice Milk (Unsweetened)
  - Serving Size: 1 cup (240ml)
  - Potassium: 30 mg
  - Calories: 120 kcal
  - Nutritional Information: 1g protein, 22g carbohydrates, 2.5g fat, 0g fiber
  - Medical Endorsement: Rice milk is very low in potassium and is a good option for those with kidney disease.
  - Evidence-Based Recommendations: Use in cereals, coffee, or as a base for soups and sauces.

3. Coconut Milk (Canned, Light)
  - Serving Size: 1/4 cup (60ml)
  - Potassium: 60 mg
  - Calories: 45 kcal
  - Nutritional Information: 0.5g protein, 1g carbohydrates, 4g fat, 0g fiber
  - Medical Endorsement: Light canned coconut milk is low in potassium and provides a creamy texture without high potassium levels.
  - Evidence-Based Recommendations: Ideal for use in cooking, baking, and adding to smoothies.

4. Coconut Yogurt (Unsweetened)
  - Serving Size: 1/2 cup (113g)
  - Potassium: 100 mg
  - Calories: 120 kcal

- Nutritional Information: 1g protein, 18g carbohydrates, 5g fat, 0g fiber
- Medical Endorsement: Coconut yogurt is a low-potassium alternative to regular yogurt and is often fortified with probiotics.
- Evidence-Based Recommendations: Use as a snack, in parfaits, or as a base for smoothies.

5. Soy Milk (Unsweetened)
- Serving Size: 1 cup (240ml)
- Potassium: 180 mg
- Calories: 80 kcal
- Nutritional Information: 7g protein, 4g carbohydrates, 4.5g fat, 1g fiber
- Medical Endorsement: Soy milk is relatively low in potassium and provides a good source of plant-based protein.
- Evidence-Based Recommendations: Suitable for use in cereals, coffee, and cooking.

6. Oat Milk (Unsweetened)
- Serving Size: 1 cup (240ml)
- Potassium: 180 mg
- Calories: 120 kcal
- Nutritional Information: 3g protein, 16g carbohydrates, 5g fat, 2g fiber

- Medical Endorsement: Oat milk is low in potassium and is often fortified with vitamins and minerals, making it a suitable dairy alternative.
- Evidence-Based Recommendations: Use in baking, smoothies, or as a milk substitute.

7. Hemp Milk (Unsweetened)
- Serving Size: 1 cup (240ml)
- Potassium: 20 mg
- Calories: 70 kcal
- Nutritional Information: 2g protein, 1g carbohydrates, 5g fat, 0g fiber
- Medical Endorsement: Hemp milk is very low in potassium and provides omega-3 fatty acids, which are beneficial for heart health.
- Evidence-Based Recommendations: Use in cereals, smoothies, or for cooking.

8. Cashew Milk (Unsweetened)
- Serving Size: 1 cup (240ml)
- Potassium: 160 mg
- Calories: 25 kcal
- Nutritional Information: 0.5g protein, 1g carbohydrates, 2g fat, 0g fiber
- Medical Endorsement: Cashew milk is a low-potassium, creamy alternative to

cow's milk and is often fortified with vitamins.

- Evidence-Based Recommendations: Ideal for use in cereals, coffee, or smoothies.

9. Coconut Cream

- Serving Size: 1 tablespoon (15ml)
- Potassium: 30 mg
- Calories: 60 kcal
- Nutritional Information: 0.6g protein, 2g carbohydrates, 6g fat, 0g fiber
- Medical Endorsement: Coconut cream is low in potassium and can be used to add richness to dishes without high potassium levels.
- Evidence-Based Recommendations: Use in curries, desserts, or as a topping.

10. Almond Yogurt (Unsweetened)

- Serving Size: 1/2 cup (113g)
- Potassium: 150 mg
- Calories: 80 kcal
- Nutritional Information: 1g protein, 12g carbohydrates, 3.5g fat, 0g fiber
- Medical Endorsement: Almond yogurt is low in potassium and is often fortified with calcium and probiotics.
- Evidence-Based Recommendations: Enjoy as a snack, with fruit, or as a base for smoothies.

11. Macadamia Milk (Unsweetened)
- Serving Size: 1 cup (240ml)
- Potassium: 120 mg
- Calories: 50 kcal
- Nutritional Information: 1g protein, 1g carbohydrates, 5g fat, 0g fiber
- Medical Endorsement: Macadamia milk is low in potassium and provides a creamy texture with a rich taste.
- Evidence-Based Recommendations: Use in cereals, coffee, or as a milk substitute in recipes.

12. Flax Milk (Unsweetened)
- Serving Size: 1 cup (240ml)
- Potassium: 60 mg
- Calories: 25 kcal
- Nutritional Information: 0g protein, 1g carbohydrates, 2.5g fat, 0g fiber
- Medical Endorsement: Flax milk is low in potassium and contains omega-3 fatty acids, which are beneficial for heart health.
- Evidence-Based Recommendations: Use in smoothies, cereals, or as a dairy alternative in recipes.

13. Coconut Water (Small Amounts)
   - Serving Size: 1/4 cup (60ml)
   - Potassium: 60 mg
   - Calories: 11 kcal
   - Nutritional Information: 0g protein, 3g carbohydrates, 0g fat, 0g fiber
   - Medical Endorsement: While coconut water contains potassium, in small amounts, it can be included as a low-potassium option.
   - Evidence-Based Recommendations: Use sparingly in smoothies or as a refreshing drink.

14. Pea Protein Milk (Unsweetened)
   - Serving Size: 1 cup (240ml)
   - Potassium: 110 mg
   - Calories: 70 kcal
   - Nutritional Information: 8g protein, 1g carbohydrates, 4.5g fat, 0g fiber
   - Medical Endorsement: Pea protein milk is low in potassium and provides a good source of plant-based protein.
   - Evidence-Based Recommendations: Suitable for use in smoothies, cereals, or as a milk substitute.

15. Quinoa Milk
   - Serving Size: 1 cup (240ml)
   - Potassium: 60 mg
   - Calories: 70 kcal

- Nutritional Information: 1g protein, 12g carbohydrates, 2.5g fat, 1g fiber
- Medical Endorsement: Quinoa milk is low in potassium and provides a slight nutty flavor with added nutrients.
- Evidence-Based Recommendations: Use in cereals, coffee, or as a milk alternative in cooking.

Herbs and spices

1. Basil
   - Serving Size: 1 tablespoon (2.6g, fresh)
   - Potassium: 10 mg
   - Calories: 1 kcal
   - Nutritional Information: 0.2g protein, 0.1g carbohydrates, 0g fat, 0.1g fiber
   - Medical Endorsement: Basil is a low-potassium herb that adds flavor without added salt.
   - Evidence-Based Recommendations: Use in salads, sauces, or as a garnish for cooked dishes.

2. Oregano
   - Serving Size: 1 teaspoon (1g, dried)
   - Potassium: 19 mg
   - Calories: 3 kcal
   - Nutritional Information: 0.1g protein, 0.7g carbohydrates, 0.1g fat, 0.4g fiber

- Medical Endorsement: Oregano is low in potassium and rich in antioxidants, making it a healthy seasoning choice.
- Evidence-Based Recommendations: Ideal for use in Mediterranean dishes, pizza, and pasta sauces.

3. Parsley

- Serving Size: 1 tablespoon (3.8g, fresh)
- Potassium: 21 mg
- Calories: 1 kcal
- Nutritional Information: 0.1g protein, 0.2g carbohydrates, 0g fat, 0.1g fiber
- Medical Endorsement: Parsley is a low-potassium herb that provides vitamin K and can enhance the flavor of dishes.
- Evidence-Based Recommendations: Use as a garnish or in salads, soups, and stews.

4. Rosemary

- Serving Size: 1 teaspoon (1g, dried)
- Potassium: 9 mg
- Calories: 2 kcal
- Nutritional Information: 0.1g protein, 0.3g carbohydrates, 0.1g fat, 0.2g fiber
- Medical Endorsement: Rosemary is low in potassium and contains anti-inflammatory compounds.

- Evidence-Based Recommendations: Use in roasted vegetables, meats, and soups.

5. Thyme
    - Serving Size: 1 teaspoon (1g, dried)
    - Potassium: 5 mg
    - Calories: 3 kcal
    - Nutritional Information: 0.1g protein, 0.7g carbohydrates, 0.1g fat, 0.4g fiber
    - Medical Endorsement: Thyme is low in potassium and has antimicrobial properties, making it a healthy addition to meals.
    - Evidence-Based Recommendations: Use in soups, stews, and marinades.

6. Cilantro
    - Serving Size: 1 tablespoon (1g, fresh)
    - Potassium: 4 mg
    - Calories: 0 kcal
    - Nutritional Information: 0.1g protein, 0.1g carbohydrates, 0g fat, 0.1g fiber
    - Medical Endorsement: Cilantro is very low in potassium and can add a fresh flavor to dishes without the need for salt.
    - Evidence-Based Recommendations: Use in salads, salsas, and as a garnish for various dishes.

7. Dill
- Serving Size: 1 tablespoon (2.1g, fresh)
- Potassium: 16 mg
- Calories: 1 kcal
- Nutritional Information: 0.2g protein, 0.2g carbohydrates, 0g fat, 0.1g fiber
- Medical Endorsement: Dill is low in potassium and can be used to enhance the flavor of food without added sodium.
- Evidence-Based Recommendations: Ideal for seasoning fish, vegetables, and salads.

8. Mint
- Serving Size: 1 tablespoon (1.6g, fresh)
- Potassium: 6 mg
- Calories: 1 kcal
- Nutritional Information: 0.1g protein, 0.3g carbohydrates, 0g fat, 0.1g fiber
- Medical Endorsement: Mint is low in potassium and can aid in digestion while providing a refreshing flavor.
- Evidence-Based Recommendations: Use in teas, salads, or as a garnish for desserts.

9. Chives
- Serving Size: 1 tablespoon (3g, fresh)
- Potassium: 9 mg
- Calories: 1 kcal

- Nutritional Information: 0.1g protein, 0.2g carbohydrates, 0g fat, 0.1g fiber
- Medical Endorsement: Chives are low in potassium and provide a mild onion-like flavor that can enhance various dishes.
- Evidence-Based Recommendations: Use in baked potatoes, salads, and as a garnish.

10. Bay Leaves
- Serving Size: 1 leaf (0.6g, dried)
- Potassium: 4 mg
- Calories: 1 kcal
- Nutritional Information: 0.1g protein, 0.2g carbohydrates, 0g fat, 0g fiber
- Medical Endorsement: Bay leaves are low in potassium and can be used to add depth of flavor to soups and stews.
- Evidence-Based Recommendations: Use in slow-cooked dishes, sauces, and marinades.

11. Tarragon
- Serving Size: 1 teaspoon (0.8g, dried)
- Potassium: 10 mg
- Calories: 2 kcal
- Nutritional Information: 0.1g protein, 0.4g carbohydrates, 0.1g fat, 0.2g fiber

- Medical Endorsement: Tarragon is low in potassium and can be used to season dishes, offering a mild licorice flavor.
- Evidence-Based Recommendations: Use in chicken dishes, sauces, and salad dressings.

12. Paprika

- Serving Size: 1 teaspoon (2.3g)
- Potassium: 35 mg
- Calories: 6 kcal
- Nutritional Information: 0.3g protein, 1.2g carbohydrates, 0.3g fat, 0.8g fiber
- Medical Endorsement: Paprika is relatively low in potassium and can add color and flavor to dishes without added sodium.
- Evidence-Based Recommendations: Use in soups, stews, and as a seasoning for meats and vegetables.

13. Cinnamon

- Serving Size: 1 teaspoon (2.6g)
- Potassium: 11 mg
- Calories: 6 kcal
- Nutritional Information: 0.1g protein, 2.1g carbohydrates, 0g fat, 1.4g fiber
- Medical Endorsement: Cinnamon is low in potassium and has anti-inflammatory properties, making it a healthy seasoning option.

- Evidence-Based Recommendations: Use in baked goods, cereals, and beverages.

14. Garlic Powder

- Serving Size: 1/4 teaspoon (0.8g)
- Potassium: 37 mg
- Calories: 2 kcal
- Nutritional Information: 0.1g protein, 0.5g carbohydrates, 0g fat, 0.1g fiber
- Medical Endorsement: Garlic powder is low in potassium and can add flavor without adding sodium, making it kidney-friendly.
- Evidence-Based Recommendations: Use in soups, stews, marinades, and seasoning for meats and vegetables.

15. Ginger (Fresh)

- Serving Size: 1 teaspoon (2g, fresh)
- Potassium: 10 mg
- Calories: 2 kcal
- Nutritional Information: 0.1g protein, 0.5g carbohydrates, 0g fat, 0.1g fiber
- Medical Endorsement: Fresh ginger is low in potassium and offers anti-inflammatory and digestive benefits.
- Evidence-Based Recommendations: Use in teas, stir-fries, and baked goods.

Vegetables

1. Cabbage
    - Serving Size: 1/2 cup (75g, cooked)
    - Potassium: 150 mg
    - Calories: 17 kcal
    - Nutritional Information: 1g protein, 4g carbohydrates, 0g fat, 1.5g fiber
    - Medical Endorsement: Cabbage is low in potassium and is a good source of vitamin C, making it a kidney-friendly vegetable.
    - Evidence-Based Recommendations: Use in salads, soups, or as a side dish.

2. Cauliflower
    - Serving Size: 1/2 cup (62g, cooked)
    - Potassium: 88 mg
    - Calories: 14 kcal
    - Nutritional Information: 1g protein, 3g carbohydrates, 0g fat, 1g fiber
    - Medical Endorsement: Cauliflower is low in potassium and rich in vitamins C and K, making it suitable for a kidney-friendly diet.
    - Evidence-Based Recommendations: Use in stir-fries, mashed as a potato substitute, or roasted.

3. Green Beans
  - Serving Size: 1/2 cup (60g, cooked)
  - Potassium: 90 mg
  - Calories: 16 kcal
  - Nutritional Information: 1g protein, 3.5g carbohydrates, 0g fat, 1.5g fiber
  - Medical Endorsement: Green beans are low in potassium and provide fiber and vitamins A and C.
  - Evidence-Based Recommendations: Serve steamed, in salads, or as a side dish.

4. Lettuce (Iceberg)
  - Serving Size: 1 cup (47g, chopped)
  - Potassium: 78 mg
  - Calories: 8 kcal
  - Nutritional Information: 0.5g protein, 1.6g carbohydrates, 0.1g fat, 0.7g fiber
  - Medical Endorsement: Iceberg lettuce is very low in potassium and can be a base for kidney-friendly salads.
  - Evidence-Based Recommendations: Use in salads, sandwiches, or as a garnish.

5. Zucchini
   - Serving Size: 1/2 cup (90g, cooked)
   - Potassium: 160 mg
   - Calories: 15 kcal
   - Nutritional Information: 1g protein, 3g carbohydrates, 0g fat, 1g fiber
   - Medical Endorsement: Zucchini is low in potassium and provides vitamin C and fiber.
   - Evidence-Based Recommendations: Use in stir-fries, grilled, or in salads.

6. Cucumber
   - Serving Size: 1/2 cup (52g, sliced)
   - Potassium: 76 mg
   - Calories: 8 kcal
   - Nutritional Information: 0.3g protein, 2g carbohydrates, 0.1g fat, 0.3g fiber
   - Medical Endorsement: Cucumbers are low in potassium and hydrating, making them a refreshing choice for kidney-friendly diets.
   - Evidence-Based Recommendations: Use in salads, sandwiches, or as a snack.

7. Bell Peppers (Green)
   - Serving Size: 1/2 cup (75g, chopped)
   - Potassium: 130 mg
   - Calories: 15 kcal

- Nutritional Information: 0.5g protein, 3g carbohydrates, 0g fat, 1g fiber
- Medical Endorsement: Green bell peppers are low in potassium and high in vitamins A and C.
- Evidence-Based Recommendations: Use in salads, stir-fries, or as a snack.

8. Eggplant

- Serving Size: 1/2 cup (49g, cooked)
- Potassium: 119 mg
- Calories: 10 kcal
- Nutritional Information: 0.2g protein, 2.4g carbohydrates, 0.1g fat, 1.3g fiber
- Medical Endorsement: Eggplant is low in potassium and can be used as a versatile ingredient in various dishes.
- Evidence-Based Recommendations: Use in stews, grilled, or as a meat substitute in recipes.

9. Radishes

- Serving Size: 1/2 cup (58g, sliced)
- Potassium: 135 mg
- Calories: 9 kcal
- Nutritional Information: 0.5g protein, 2g carbohydrates, 0g fat, 1g fiber
- Medical Endorsement: Radishes are low in potassium and offer a crunchy texture and peppery flavor.

- Evidence-Based Recommendations: Use in salads, as a garnish, or as a snack.

10. Onion (Yellow)
    - Serving Size: 1/2 cup (58g, cooked)
    - Potassium: 116 mg
    - Calories: 32 kcal
    - Nutritional Information: 0.8g protein, 7.5g carbohydrates, 0.1g fat, 1g fiber
    - Medical Endorsement: Yellow onions are low in potassium and can be used to add flavor to various dishes without added salt.
    - Evidence-Based Recommendations: Use in soups, stews, or as a base for cooking.

11. Kale
    - Serving Size: 1/2 cup (34g, cooked)
    - Potassium: 148 mg
    - Calories: 18 kcal
    - Nutritional Information: 1g protein, 3.4g carbohydrates, 0.3g fat, 1g fiber
    - Medical Endorsement: Kale is low in potassium and high in vitamins A, C, and K, making it a nutrient-dense option.
    - Evidence-Based Recommendations: Use in salads, smoothies, or lightly steamed as a side dish.

12. Turnips

- Serving Size: 1/2 cup (78g, cooked)
- Potassium: 140 mg
- Calories: 17 kcal
- Nutritional Information: 0.6g protein, 4g carbohydrates, 0g fat, 1.6g fiber
- Medical Endorsement: Turnips are low in potassium and provide fiber and vitamin C.
- Evidence-Based Recommendations: Use in soups, stews, or mashed as a potato substitute.

13. Carrots

- Serving Size: 1/2 cup (61g, cooked)
- Potassium: 180 mg
- Calories: 25 kcal
- Nutritional Information: 0.6g protein, 6g carbohydrates, 0.1g fat, 1.8g fiber
- Medical Endorsement: Carrots are low in potassium and are an excellent source of beta-carotene.
- Evidence-Based Recommendations: Use in salads, soups, or as a side dish.

14. Bok Choy

- Serving Size: 1/2 cup (85g, cooked)
- Potassium: 176 mg
- Calories: 10 kcal
- Nutritional Information: 1g protein, 2g carbohydrates, 0.1g fat, 0.7g fiber

- Medical Endorsement: Bok choy is low in potassium and rich in vitamins A, C, and K.
- Evidence-Based Recommendations: Use in stir-fries, soups, or as a steamed side dish.

15. Asparagus
    - Serving Size: 4 spears (60g, cooked)
    - Potassium: 115 mg
    - Calories: 13 kcal
    - Nutritional Information: 1.5g protein, 2.5g carbohydrates, 0g fat, 1.5g fiber
    - Medical Endorsement: Asparagus is low in potassium and provides fiber and folate.
    - Evidence-Based Recommendations: Use in salads, stir-fries, or as a side dish.

Grains

1. White Rice
   - Serving Size: 1/2 cup (79g, cooked)
   - Potassium: 28 mg
   - Calories: 103 kcal
   - Nutritional Information: 2.1g protein, 22.3g carbohydrates, 0.2g fat, 0.3g fiber
   - Medical Endorsement: White rice is low in potassium and easily digestible, making it a staple in kidney-friendly diets.
   - Evidence-Based Recommendations: Use as a base for meals or in soups and casseroles.

2. Couscous
   - Serving Size: 1/2 cup (125g, cooked)
   - Potassium: 55 mg
   - Calories: 88 kcal
   - Nutritional Information: 3g protein, 18g carbohydrates, 0.2g fat, 1g fiber
   - Medical Endorsement: Couscous is low in potassium and provides a good source of carbohydrates for energy.
   - Evidence-Based Recommendations: Use as a side dish or as a base for salads and main dishes.

3. Polenta (Cornmeal)
- Serving Size: 1/2 cup (125g, cooked)
- Potassium: 20 mg
- Calories: 73 kcal
- Nutritional Information: 2g protein, 15g carbohydrates, 0.2g fat, 1g fiber
- Medical Endorsement: Polenta is low in potassium and is a versatile grain option that can be used in various dishes.
- Evidence-Based Recommendations: Serve as a side dish, in casseroles, or as a base for toppings.

4. Pasta (Regular)
- Serving Size: 1/2 cup (70g, cooked)
- Potassium: 37 mg
- Calories: 111 kcal
- Nutritional Information: 4g protein, 22g carbohydrates, 0.6g fat, 1g fiber
- Medical Endorsement: Regular pasta is low in potassium and a good source of energy for those with kidney disease.
- Evidence-Based Recommendations: Use as a base for pasta dishes or in soups and salads.

5. Tortillas (Corn)
- Serving Size: 1 tortilla (24g)
- Potassium: 37 mg
- Calories: 52 kcal

- Nutritional Information: 1g protein, 11g carbohydrates, 0.7g fat, 1g fiber
- Medical Endorsement: Corn tortillas are low in potassium and can be a good alternative to bread for those on a kidney-friendly diet.
- Evidence-Based Recommendations: Use for wraps, tacos, or as a side to main dishes.

6. Grits

- Serving Size: 1/2 cup (120g, cooked)
- Potassium: 40 mg
- Calories: 109 kcal
- Nutritional Information: 2.5g protein, 23g carbohydrates, 0.6g fat, 0.6g fiber
- Medical Endorsement: Grits are low in potassium and provide a warm, comforting meal option for breakfast or dinner.
- Evidence-Based Recommendations: Serve as a breakfast dish or as a side to savory meals.

7. Oatmeal

- Serving Size: 1/2 cup (117g, cooked)
- Potassium: 80 mg
- Calories: 77 kcal
- Nutritional Information: 3g protein, 13g carbohydrates, 1.5g fat, 1.5g fiber

- Medical Endorsement: Oatmeal is relatively low in potassium and offers a heart-healthy option with soluble fiber.
- Evidence-Based Recommendations: Serve for breakfast with low-potassium fruits or as a snack.

8. Barley (Pearled)
- Serving Size: 1/2 cup (78g, cooked)
- Potassium: 54 mg
- Calories: 97 kcal
- Nutritional Information: 2g protein, 22g carbohydrates, 0.3g fat, 3g fiber
- Medical Endorsement: Pearled barley is low in potassium and provides dietary fiber, making it a healthy grain option.
- Evidence-Based Recommendations: Use in soups, stews, or as a side dish.

9. Rice Noodles
- Serving Size: 1 cup (176g, cooked)
- Potassium: 30 mg
- Calories: 192 kcal
- Nutritional Information: 3g protein, 43g carbohydrates, 0.4g fat, 1g fiber
- Medical Endorsement: Rice noodles are low in potassium and can be a good substitute for traditional pasta.
- Evidence-Based Recommendations: Use in stir-fries, soups, or as a base for noodle dishes.

10. Quinoa
- Serving Size: 1/2 cup (92g, cooked)
- Potassium: 159 mg
- Calories: 111 kcal
- Nutritional Information: 4g protein, 20g carbohydrates, 1.8g fat, 2.5g fiber
- Medical Endorsement: Quinoa is relatively low in potassium and provides a complete source of protein and fiber.
- Evidence-Based Recommendations: Use as a side dish, in salads, or as a base for main dishes.

11. Farro
- Serving Size: 1/2 cup (84g, cooked)
- Potassium: 95 mg
- Calories: 100 kcal
- Nutritional Information: 4g protein, 20g carbohydrates, 0.5g fat, 3g fiber
- Medical Endorsement: Farro is low in potassium and a good source of protein and fiber, suitable for a kidney-friendly diet.
- Evidence-Based Recommendations: Use in salads, soups, or as a side dish.

12. Millet
- Serving Size: 1/2 cup (84g, cooked)
- Potassium: 52 mg
- Calories: 103 kcal

- Nutritional Information: 3g protein, 21g carbohydrates, 0.5g fat, 1g fiber
- Medical Endorsement: Millet is low in potassium and gluten-free, making it a versatile grain option for those with CKD.
- Evidence-Based Recommendations: Use as a side dish, in salads, or as a base for grain bowls.

13. White Bread

- Serving Size: 1 slice (25g)
- Potassium: 30 mg
- Calories: 67 kcal
- Nutritional Information: 1.9g protein, 13g carbohydrates, 0.8g fat, 0.5g fiber
- Medical Endorsement: White bread is low in potassium and often recommended as a staple for kidney-friendly diets.
- Evidence-Based Recommendations: Use for sandwiches, toast, or as a side to meals.

14. Rice Cakes

- Serving Size: 1 rice cake (9g)
- Potassium: 17 mg
- Calories: 35 kcal
- Nutritional Information: 0.7g protein, 7.3g carbohydrates, 0.3g fat, 0.2g fiber

- Medical Endorsement: Rice cakes are low in potassium and can be a crunchy, light snack option.
- Evidence-Based Recommendations: Use as a snack with low-potassium toppings or as a base for light meals.

15. Bulgur
    - Serving Size: 1/2 cup (91g, cooked)
    - Potassium: 62 mg
    - Calories: 76 kcal
    - Nutritional Information: 3g protein, 17g carbohydrates, 0.2g fat, 4g fiber
    - Medical Endorsement: Bulgur is low in potassium and high in fiber, making it a heart-healthy and kidney-friendly grain option.
    - Evidence-Based Recommendations: Use in salads, pilafs, or as a side dish.

1. Chicken Breast (Skinless, Boneless)
- Serving Size: 3 oz (85g, cooked)
- Potassium: 220 mg
- Calories: 140 kcal
- Nutritional Information: 26g protein, 0g carbohydrates, 3g fat
- Medical Endorsement: Chicken breast is low in potassium and a lean protein source, suitable for a kidney-friendly diet.
- Evidence-Based Recommendations: Opt for grilled or baked preparation without added salt.

2. Turkey Breast (Skinless, Boneless)
- Serving Size: 3 oz (85g, cooked)
- Potassium: 250 mg
- Calories: 135 kcal
- Nutritional Information: 25g protein, 0g carbohydrates, 3g fat
- Medical Endorsement: Turkey breast is a low-potassium, lean protein that supports muscle maintenance in seniors.
- Evidence-Based Recommendations: Use in sandwiches, salads, or as a main dish.

3. Egg Whites

- Serving Size: 2 large egg whites (66g)
- Potassium: 108 mg
- Calories: 34 kcal
- Nutritional Information: 7g protein, 0.6g carbohydrates, 0g fat
- Medical Endorsement: Egg whites are very low in potassium and an excellent source of high-quality protein.
- Evidence-Based Recommendations: Incorporate into omelets, scrambles, or as a protein supplement.

4. Tilapia

- Serving Size: 3 oz (85g, cooked)
- Potassium: 340 mg
- Calories: 110 kcal
- Nutritional Information: 22g protein, 0g carbohydrates, 2.3g fat
- Medical Endorsement: Tilapia is a low-potassium fish option rich in protein and essential omega-3 fatty acids.
- Evidence-Based Recommendations: Grill or bake with herbs and spices, avoiding salt-based seasonings.

5. Ground Turkey (Lean)

- Serving Size: 3 oz (85g, cooked)
- Potassium: 244 mg
- Calories: 120 kcal

- Nutritional Information: 21g protein, 0g carbohydrates, 3g fat
- Medical Endorsement: Lean ground turkey provides a good protein source with low potassium content.
- Evidence-Based Recommendations: Use in burgers, meatloaf, or tacos with low-potassium toppings.

6. Cottage Cheese (Low-Sodium)

- Serving Size: 1/2 cup (113g)
- Potassium: 104 mg
- Calories: 81 kcal
- Nutritional Information: 14g protein, 3g carbohydrates, 2g fat
- Medical Endorsement: Low-sodium cottage cheese is low in potassium and offers a convenient protein source.
- Evidence-Based Recommendations: Pair with low-potassium fruits or vegetables for a balanced snack.

7. Tuna (Canned in Water, Drained)

- Serving Size: 3 oz (85g)
- Potassium: 130 mg
- Calories: 99 kcal
- Nutritional Information: 20g protein, 0g carbohydrates, 0.7g fat
- Medical Endorsement: Canned tuna is low in potassium and provides lean protein with minimal fat.

- Evidence-Based Recommendations: Use in salads, sandwiches, or mixed with low-potassium vegetables.

8. Cod

- Serving Size: 3 oz (85g, cooked)
- Potassium: 324 mg
- Calories: 70 kcal
- Nutritional Information: 15g protein, 0g carbohydrates, 0.5g fat
- Medical Endorsement: Cod is low in potassium and provides a lean, healthy source of protein.
- Evidence-Based Recommendations: Best when grilled or baked with herbs, avoiding salty sauces.

9. Pork Loin (Lean)

- Serving Size: 3 oz (85g, cooked)
- Potassium: 360 mg
- Calories: 206 kcal
- Nutritional Information: 23g protein, 0g carbohydrates, 12g fat
- Medical Endorsement: Lean pork loin is a low-potassium protein that can be part of a balanced diet.
- Evidence-Based Recommendations: Serve as a main dish, using low-sodium marinades and spices.

10. Greek Yogurt (Plain, Low-Sodium)
   - Serving Size: 1/2 cup (113g)
   - Potassium: 141 mg
   - Calories: 59 kcal
   - Nutritional Information: 10g protein, 4g carbohydrates, 0.5g fat
   - Medical Endorsement: Low-sodium Greek yogurt is relatively low in potassium and offers high protein content.
   - Evidence-Based Recommendations: Use as a snack or in recipes, choosing unsweetened varieties.

11. Scallops
   - Serving Size: 3 oz (85g, cooked)
   - Potassium: 322 mg
   - Calories: 94 kcal
   - Nutritional Information: 17g protein, 0g carbohydrates, 1g fat
   - Medical Endorsement: Scallops are low in potassium and provide lean, high-quality protein.
   - Evidence-Based Recommendations: Best served grilled or seared with low-potassium herbs and spices.

12. Salmon (Wild-Caught)
   - Serving Size: 3 oz (85g, cooked)
   - Potassium: 326 mg
   - Calories: 175 kcal

- Nutritional Information: 18g protein, 0g carbohydrates, 10g fat
- Medical Endorsement: Wild-caught salmon is low in potassium and rich in omega-3 fatty acids.
- Evidence-Based Recommendations: Grill or bake, using low-potassium seasonings to enhance flavor.

13. Chicken Thigh (Skinless, Boneless)
   - Serving Size: 3 oz (85g, cooked)
   - Potassium: 212 mg
   - Calories: 209 kcal
   - Nutritional Information: 19g protein, 0g carbohydrates, 14g fat
   - Medical Endorsement: Chicken thigh provides a low-potassium protein option, though slightly higher in fat.
   - Evidence-Based Recommendations: Best when baked or grilled, paired with low-potassium sides.

14. Tempeh
   - Serving Size: 1/2 cup (126g)
   - Potassium: 221 mg
   - Calories: 160 kcal
   - Nutritional Information: 15g protein, 9g carbohydrates, 9g fat
   - Medical Endorsement: Tempeh is a low-potassium plant-based protein, rich in fiber and nutrients.

- Evidence-Based Recommendations: Use in stir-fries, salads, or as a meat substitute.

15. Tofu (Firm)
   - Serving Size: 3 oz (85g)
   - Potassium: 121 mg
   - Calories: 70 kcal
   - Nutritional Information: 8g protein, 2g carbohydrates, 4g fat
   - Medical Endorsement: Firm tofu is low in potassium and offers a versatile plant-based protein option.
   - Evidence-Based Recommendations: Use in a variety of dishes, such as stir-fries or grilled as a meat substitute.

Snacks

1. Unsalted Popcorn
- Serving Size: 3 cups (24g, air-popped)
- Potassium: 60 mg
- Calories: 93 kcal
- Nutritional Information: 3g protein, 19g carbohydrates, 1.1g fat, 3.6g fiber
- Medical Endorsement: Unsalted popcorn is low in potassium and a good source of fiber, making it a healthy snack option.
- Evidence-Based Recommendations: Enjoy plain or with a sprinkle of herb-based seasonings.

2. Apple Slices
- Serving Size: 1 medium apple (182g)
- Potassium: 195 mg
- Calories: 95 kcal
- Nutritional Information: 0.5g protein, 25g carbohydrates, 0.3g fat, 4.4g fiber
- Medical Endorsement: Apples are low in potassium and provide a good source of fiber and vitamin C.
- Evidence-Based Recommendations: Pair with a small amount of peanut butter or cheese for added protein.

3. Rice Cakes with Jam
- Serving Size: 1 rice cake (9g) + 1 tbsp jam (20g)
- Potassium: 22 mg
- Calories: 70 kcal
- Nutritional Information: 0.5g protein, 16g carbohydrates, 0g fat, 0.2g fiber
- Medical Endorsement: Rice cakes are low in potassium and can be topped with low-potassium spreads for a quick snack.
- Evidence-Based Recommendations: Choose unsweetened jam or jelly to reduce added sugar intake.

4. Graham Crackers
- Serving Size: 2 squares (31g)
- Potassium: 60 mg
- Calories: 130 kcal
- Nutritional Information: 2g protein, 24g carbohydrates, 3g fat, 1g fiber
- Medical Endorsement: Graham crackers are low in potassium and provide a sweet, crunchy snack option.
- Evidence-Based Recommendations: Enjoy with a small amount of cream cheese or as is for a light treat.

5. Blueberry Muffin (Low Sodium)
- Serving Size: 1 small muffin (55g)
- Potassium: 55 mg
- Calories: 187 kcal
- Nutritional Information: 3g protein, 27g carbohydrates, 7g fat, 1g fiber
- Medical Endorsement: A low-sodium blueberry muffin is low in potassium and provides a sweet snack without excessive sodium.
- Evidence-Based Recommendations: Look for low-sodium recipes or store-bought options to keep sodium levels in check.

6. Cucumber Slices with Cream Cheese
- Serving Size: 1/2 cup cucumber slices (52g) + 1 tbsp cream cheese (14g)
- Potassium: 50 mg
- Calories: 58 kcal
- Nutritional Information: 1g protein, 3g carbohydrates, 5g fat, 0.3g fiber
- Medical Endorsement: Cucumbers are low in potassium, and when paired with cream cheese, they offer a light and refreshing snack.
- Evidence-Based Recommendations: Use low-fat cream cheese to reduce calorie intake if necessary.

7. Rice Pudding (Low-Sodium)
- Serving Size: 1/2 cup (130g)
- Potassium: 60 mg
- Calories: 150 kcal
- Nutritional Information: 3g protein, 28g carbohydrates, 2g fat, 1g fiber
- Medical Endorsement: Rice pudding made with low-sodium ingredients is low in potassium and provides a comforting, sweet snack.
- Evidence-Based Recommendations: Opt for homemade versions to control potassium and sodium levels.

8. Pineapple Chunks
- Serving Size: 1/2 cup (82g)
- Potassium: 88 mg
- Calories: 41 kcal
- Nutritional Information: 0.4g protein, 10.7g carbohydrates, 0.1g fat, 1.2g fiber
- Medical Endorsement: Pineapple is low in potassium and high in vitamin C, making it a refreshing fruit option.
- Evidence-Based Recommendations: Enjoy fresh or canned in its own juice without added sugars.

9. Hard-Boiled Egg
- Serving Size: 1 large egg (50g)
- Potassium: 63 mg
- Calories: 78 kcal

- Nutritional Information: 6g protein, 0.6g carbohydrates, 5g fat
- Medical Endorsement: Hard-boiled eggs are low in potassium and provide a high-quality protein source.
- Evidence-Based Recommendations: Keep on hand for a quick, protein-rich snack.

10. Unsalted Almonds
   - Serving Size: 10 almonds (14g)
   - Potassium: 36 mg
   - Calories: 82 kcal
   - Nutritional Information: 3g protein, 3g carbohydrates, 7g fat, 1.5g fiber
   - Medical Endorsement: Unsalted almonds are low in potassium and offer healthy fats and protein.
   - Evidence-Based Recommendations: Enjoy a small handful as a satisfying and nutrient-dense snack.

11. Apple Sauce (Unsweetened)
   - Serving Size: 1/2 cup (122g)
   - Potassium: 90 mg
   - Calories: 51 kcal
   - Nutritional Information: 0.1g protein, 13g carbohydrates, 0g fat, 1.5g fiber
   - Medical Endorsement: Unsweetened apple sauce is low in potassium and free

of added sugars, making it a healthy snack option.
- Evidence-Based Recommendations: Pair with a sprinkle of cinnamon for added flavor.

12. Rice Crisps
- Serving Size: 1 oz (28g)
- Potassium: 40 mg
- Calories: 110 kcal
- Nutritional Information: 2g protein, 23g carbohydrates, 1g fat, 1g fiber
- Medical Endorsement: Rice crisps are low in potassium and provide a crunchy, satisfying snack option.
- Evidence-Based Recommendations: Choose plain or lightly flavored varieties without added sodium.

13. Carrot Sticks with Hummus
- Serving Size: 1/2 cup carrot sticks (61g) + 2 tbsp hummus (30g)
- Potassium: 190 mg
- Calories: 105 kcal
- Nutritional Information: 2g protein, 13g carbohydrates, 6g fat, 3g fiber
- Medical Endorsement: Carrots are relatively low in potassium, and when paired with hummus, they offer a nutrient-rich snack.

- Evidence-Based Recommendations: Use a low-potassium hummus to keep the potassium content manageable.

14. Mini Rice Crackers
   - Serving Size: 1 oz (28g)
   - Potassium: 30 mg
   - Calories: 120 kcal
   - Nutritional Information: 2g protein, 24g carbohydrates, 2g fat, 1g fiber
   - Medical Endorsement: Mini rice crackers are low in potassium and provide a light, crunchy snack option.
   - Evidence-Based Recommendations: Pair with low-potassium dips like Greek yogurt or cream cheese.

15. Watermelon Cubes
   - Serving Size: 1 cup (152g)
   - Potassium: 170 mg
   - Calories: 46 kcal
   - Nutritional Information: 0.9g protein, 11.5g carbohydrates, 0.2g fat, 0.6g fiber
   - Medical Endorsement: Watermelon is low in potassium and high in water content, making it a hydrating snack.
   - Evidence-Based Recommendations: Enjoy fresh or in fruit salads, but monitor portion size to control potassium intake.

30 HEALTHY AND EASY KIDNEY FRIENDLY RECIPES FOR SENIORS ON STAGE 4

Breakfast Recipes

1. Apple Cinnamon Oatmeal

Ingredients:
1. 1/2 cup old-fashioned oats
2. 1 cup water
3. 1/2 cup unsweetened applesauce
4. 1/2 tsp ground cinnamon
5. 1 tsp honey (optional)
6. 1 tbsp chopped walnuts (optional)

Preparation:
1. In a small pot, bring the water to a boil.
2. Add the oats and reduce the heat to medium. Cook for about 5 minutes, stirring occasionally.
3. Stir in the applesauce and cinnamon. Cook for an additional 2 minutes.
4. Remove from heat and top with honey and walnuts if desired.
5. Prep Time: 10 minutes

Nutritional Information (Per Serving):
- Calories: 180 kcal
- Potassium: 160 mg
- Phosphorus: 110 mg
- Sodium: 5 mg
- Protein: 4g
- Carbohydrates: 34g
- Fat: 3g
- Fiber: 4g

2. Low-Sodium Scrambled Eggs with Bell Peppers

Ingredients:
1. 2 large eggs
2. 1/4 cup diced bell peppers (red or green)
3. 1 tbsp unsalted butter or olive oil
4. Ground black pepper (to taste)
5. Fresh parsley for garnish

Preparation:
1. Heat the butter or oil in a non-stick skillet over medium heat.
2. Add the diced bell peppers and sauté until slightly softened, about 3 minutes.
3. Beat the eggs in a bowl and pour them into the skillet with the peppers.

4. Cook, stirring frequently, until the eggs are fully scrambled and cooked through.
5. Season with black pepper and garnish with fresh parsley.
6. Prep Time: 10 minutes

Nutritional Information (Per Serving):
- Calories: 150 kcal
- Potassium: 120 mg
- Phosphorus: 150 mg
- Sodium: 60 mg
- Protein: 12g
- Carbohydrates: 2g
- Fat: 11g
- Fiber: 0.5g

3. Berry Smoothie Bowl

Ingredients:
1. 1/2 cup frozen mixed berries (blueberries, strawberries, raspberries)
2. 1/2 cup almond milk (unsweetened)
3. 1/4 cup low-potassium vanilla yogurt
4. 1 tbsp chia seeds
5. 1 tbsp sliced almonds (optional)
6. Fresh mint for garnish

Preparation:

1. In a blender, combine the frozen berries, almond milk, and yogurt. Blend until smooth.
2. Pour the smoothie into a bowl and top with chia seeds and sliced almonds.
3. Garnish with fresh mint and serve immediately.
4. Prep Time: 5 minutes

Nutritional Information (Per Serving):
- Calories: 160 kcal
- Potassium: 170 mg
- Phosphorus: 70 mg
- Sodium: 50 mg
- Protein: 5g
- Carbohydrates: 22g
- Fat: 6g
- Fiber: 7g

4. Cinnamon Raisin Toast with Almond Butter

Ingredients:
1. 1 slice low-sodium cinnamon raisin bread
2. 1 tbsp almond butter (unsalted)
3. 1/4 tsp ground cinnamon (optional)
4. 1/2 tsp honey (optional)

Preparation:

1. Toast the cinnamon raisin bread until golden brown.
2. Spread almond butter evenly over the toast.
3. Sprinkle with ground cinnamon and drizzle with honey if desired.
4. Prep Time: 5 minutes

Nutritional Information (Per Serving):
- Calories: 190 kcal
- Potassium: 120 mg
- Phosphorus: 100 mg
- Sodium: 50 mg
- Protein: 5g
- Carbohydrates: 22g
- Fat: 9g
- Fiber: 3g

5. Veggie Breakfast Wrap

Ingredients:
1. 1 whole wheat tortilla (low sodium)
2. 1/4 cup diced bell peppers
3. 1/4 cup sliced mushrooms
4. 1/4 cup spinach leaves (optional, use in small amounts)
5. 1 tbsp unsalted butter or olive oil
6. 1 tbsp low-sodium, low-fat cream cheese
7. Ground black pepper (to taste)

Preparation:
1. Heat the butter or oil in a skillet over medium heat.
2. Sauté the bell peppers, mushrooms, and spinach until tender, about 3-4 minutes.
3. Spread cream cheese on the tortilla.
4. Add the sautéed vegetables, season with black pepper, and roll up the wrap.
5. Serve warm.
6. Prep Time: 15 minutes

Nutritional Information (Per Serving):
- Calories: 210 kcal
- Potassium: 180 mg
- Phosphorus: 120 mg
- Sodium: 130 mg
- Protein: 7g
- Carbohydrates: 28g
- Fat: 9g
- Fiber: 4g

1. Grilled Chicken Salad with Apples and Walnuts

Ingredients:
1. 3 oz grilled chicken breast (skinless, boneless)
2. 2 cups mixed salad greens (romaine, iceberg)
3. 1/2 apple, thinly sliced
4. 1 tbsp chopped walnuts
5. 1 tbsp olive oil
6. 1 tbsp apple cider vinegar
7. Ground black pepper (to taste)

Preparation:
1. Grill the chicken breast until fully cooked, about 5-7 minutes per side. Let it cool slightly, then slice.
2. In a large bowl, combine salad greens, apple slices, and walnuts.
3. Whisk together olive oil, apple cider vinegar, and black pepper for dressing.
4. Top the salad with sliced grilled chicken and drizzle with the dressing.
5. Serve immediately.
6. Prep Time: 20 minutes

Nutritional Information (Per Serving):
- Calories: 320 kcal
- Potassium: 350 mg
- Phosphorus: 220 mg
- Sodium: 80 mg
- Protein: 22g
- Carbohydrates: 15g
- Fat: 20g
- Fiber: 3g

2. Turkey and Cucumber Sandwich

Ingredients:
1. 2 slices low-sodium whole wheat bread
2. 3 oz low-sodium turkey breast (thinly sliced)
3. 1/4 cup cucumber slices
4. 1 tbsp low-sodium mayonnaise
5. 1 leaf of lettuce
6. Ground black pepper (to taste)

Preparation:
1. Spread mayonnaise on one slice of bread.
2. Layer the turkey, cucumber slices, and lettuce on top.
3. Season with black pepper and top with the second slice of bread.
4. Slice the sandwich in half and serve.
5. Prep Time: 10 minutes

Nutritional Information (Per Serving):
- Calories: 250 kcal
- Potassium: 240 mg
- Phosphorus: 180 mg
- Sodium: 210 mg
- Protein: 18g
- Carbohydrates: 30g
- Fat: 7g
- Fiber: 4g

3. Quinoa and Roasted Vegetable Bowl

Ingredients:
1. 1/2 cup cooked quinoa
2. 1/4 cup diced zucchini
3. 1/4 cup diced red bell pepper
4. 1/4 cup diced yellow squash
5. 1 tbsp olive oil
6. 1 tsp dried oregano
7. Ground black pepper (to taste)

Preparation:
1. Preheat the oven to 400°F (200°C).
2. Toss the zucchini, bell pepper, and yellow squash in olive oil, oregano, and black pepper.
3. Spread the vegetables on a baking sheet and roast for 15 minutes or until tender.
4. Serve the roasted vegetables over the cooked quinoa.
5. Prep Time: 25 minutes

Nutritional Information (Per Serving):
- Calories: 220 kcal
- Potassium: 290 mg
- Phosphorus: 180 mg
- Sodium: 10 mg
- Protein: 6g
- Carbohydrates: 32g
- Fat: 8g
- Fiber: 4g

4. Chicken and Rice Lettuce Wraps

Ingredients:
1. 3 oz cooked chicken breast (shredded)
2. 1/2 cup cooked white rice
3. 4 large lettuce leaves (romaine or butter lettuce)
4. 1/4 cup shredded carrots
5. 1 tbsp low-sodium soy sauce
6. 1 tbsp rice vinegar
7. 1 tsp sesame oil
8. Fresh cilantro for garnish

Preparation:
1. In a small bowl, mix together the soy sauce, rice vinegar, and sesame oil.
2. In a separate bowl, combine the shredded chicken, cooked rice, and shredded carrots.

3. Drizzle the soy sauce mixture over the chicken and rice, and mix well.
4. Spoon the mixture into the lettuce leaves and garnish with fresh cilantro.
5. Serve the lettuce wraps cold or at room temperature.
6. Prep Time: 15 minutes

Nutritional Information (Per Serving):
- Calories: 260 kcal
- Potassium: 260 mg
- Phosphorus: 200 mg
- Sodium: 180 mg
- Protein: 18g
- Carbohydrates: 28g
- Fat: 8g
- Fiber: 2g

5. Veggie and Hummus Pita

Ingredients:
1. 1 whole wheat pita (low sodium)
2. 1/4 cup hummus (low sodium)
3. 1/4 cup sliced cucumber
4. 1/4 cup sliced red bell pepper
5. 1/4 cup shredded carrots
6. 1 tbsp crumbled feta cheese (optional)
7. Fresh lemon juice (optional)

Preparation:
1. Cut the pita in half to create two pockets.
2. Spread hummus inside each pita half.
3. Fill each pita pocket with cucumber, bell pepper, and shredded carrots.
4. Add feta cheese if desired, and drizzle with a bit of fresh lemon juice.
5. Serve immediately.
6. Prep Time: 10 minutes

Nutritional Information (Per Serving):
- Calories: 290 kcal
- Potassium: 310 mg
- Phosphorus: 160 mg
- Sodium: 220 mg
- Protein: 8g
- Carbohydrates: 44g
- Fat: 10g
- Fiber: 7g

Dinner Recipes

1. Baked Herb-Crusted Cod

Ingredients:
1. 4 oz cod fillet
2. 1 tbsp olive oil
3. 1/4 cup panko breadcrumbs (unsalted)
4. 1 tsp dried thyme
5. 1 tsp dried parsley
6. 1 clove garlic, minced
7. Ground black pepper (to taste)
8. Lemon wedge (optional for serving)

Preparation:
1. Preheat oven to 375°F (190°C).
2. In a small bowl, mix together panko breadcrumbs, dried thyme, parsley, garlic, and black pepper.
3. Brush the cod fillet with olive oil and press the breadcrumb mixture onto the top of the fish.
4. Place the fillet on a baking sheet lined with parchment paper.
5. Bake for 12-15 minutes or until the fish is cooked through and the crust is golden brown.
6. Serve with a lemon wedge if desired.
7. Prep Time: 20 minutes

Nutritional Information (Per Serving):
- Calories: 230 kcal
- Potassium: 310 mg
- Phosphorus: 200 mg
- Sodium: 100 mg
- Protein: 24g
- Carbohydrates: 8g
- Fat: 10g
- Fiber: 1g

2. Stuffed Bell Peppers

Ingredients:
1. 1 medium red bell pepper, halved and seeded
2. 1/2 cup cooked quinoa
3. 2 oz ground turkey (lean)
4. 1/4 cup diced zucchini
5. 1/4 cup diced tomatoes (low sodium, drained)
6. 1 tbsp olive oil
7. 1 tsp dried basil
8. Ground black pepper (to taste)

Preparation:
1. Preheat oven to 375°F (190°C).
2. In a skillet, heat olive oil over medium heat and cook the ground turkey until browned.

3. Add diced zucchini, tomatoes, and basil to the turkey, and cook for another 3-4 minutes.
4. Stir in the cooked quinoa and season with black pepper.
5. Fill each bell pepper half with the turkey-quinoa mixture.
6. Place stuffed peppers in a baking dish and cover with foil.
7. Bake for 25-30 minutes or until the peppers are tender.
8. Prep Time: 40 minutes

Nutritional Information (Per Serving):
- Calories: 280 kcal
- Potassium: 420 mg
- Phosphorus: 230 mg
- Sodium: 150 mg
- Protein: 18g
- Carbohydrates: 28g
- Fat: 12g
- Fiber: 6g

3. Lemon Garlic Chicken with Asparagus

Ingredients:
1. 4 oz chicken breast (skinless, boneless)
2. 1/2 lb asparagus spears, trimmed
3. 1 tbsp olive oil
4. 1 clove garlic, minced

5. Juice of 1/2 lemon
6. 1 tsp dried oregano
7. Ground black pepper (to taste)

Preparation:
1. Preheat oven to 375°F (190°C).
2. In a small bowl, mix together olive oil, minced garlic, lemon juice, oregano, and black pepper.
3. Place the chicken breast and asparagus on a baking sheet lined with parchment paper.
4. Drizzle the olive oil mixture over the chicken and asparagus.
5. Bake for 20-25 minutes, or until the chicken is cooked through and the asparagus is tender.
6. Prep Time: 30 minutes

Nutritional Information (Per Serving):
- Calories: 240 kcal
- Potassium: 440 mg
- Phosphorus: 220 mg
- Sodium: 90 mg
- Protein: 26g
- Carbohydrates: 8g
- Fat: 12g
- Fiber: 4g

4. Vegetable Stir-Fry with Tofu

Ingredients:
1. 1/2 cup firm tofu, cubed
2. 1/4 cup sliced carrots
3. 1/4 cup sliced bell peppers
4. 1/4 cup broccoli florets
5. 1 tbsp low-sodium soy sauce
6. 1 tbsp sesame oil
7. 1 tsp rice vinegar
8. 1 tsp fresh ginger, minced
9. 1 clove garlic, minced
10. Fresh cilantro for garnish (optional)

Preparation:
1. Heat sesame oil in a large skillet or wok over medium-high heat.
2. Add tofu cubes and cook until golden brown on all sides, about 5 minutes.
3. Remove tofu from the skillet and set aside.
4. In the same skillet, add minced garlic and ginger, and sauté for 1 minute.
5. Add the sliced carrots, bell peppers, and broccoli, and stir-fry for 5-7 minutes.
6. Return the tofu to the skillet and add low-sodium soy sauce and rice vinegar.
7. Stir-fry for another 2-3 minutes until well combined and heated through.
8. Garnish with fresh cilantro if desired.

9. Prep Time: 20 minutes

Nutritional Information (Per Serving):
- Calories: 210 kcal
- Potassium: 380 mg
- Phosphorus: 160 mg
- Sodium: 180 mg
- Protein: 10g
- Carbohydrates: 14g
- Fat: 12g
- Fiber: 4g

5. Baked Tilapia with Roasted Veggies

Ingredients:
1. 4 oz tilapia fillet
2. 1/4 cup cherry tomatoes, halved
3. 1/2 cup zucchini, sliced
4. 1 tbsp olive oil
5. 1 tsp dried basil
6. 1/2 tsp dried thyme
7. Ground black pepper (to taste)
8. Lemon wedge (optional for serving)

Preparation:
1. Preheat oven to 375°F (190°C).
2. Place the tilapia fillet on a baking sheet lined with parchment paper.

3. Toss cherry tomatoes and zucchini slices with olive oil, dried basil, thyme, and black pepper.
4. Arrange the vegetables around the tilapia fillet on the baking sheet.
5. Bake for 12-15 minutes, or until the fish is cooked through and the vegetables are tender.
6. Serve with a lemon wedge if desired.
7. Prep Time: 25 minutes

Nutritional Information (Per Serving):
- Calories: 220 kcal
- Potassium: 420 mg
- Phosphorus: 200 mg
- Sodium: 90 mg
- Protein: 22g
- Carbohydrates: 9g
- Fat: 12g
- Fiber: 2g

1. Cucumber and Dill Greek Yogurt Dip

Ingredients:
1. 1/2 cup plain Greek yogurt (unsweetened, low-sodium)
2. 1/4 cup finely chopped cucumber (peeled and seeded)
3. 1 tsp fresh dill, chopped
4. 1 tsp lemon juice
5. Ground black pepper (to taste)
6. Raw vegetables (like bell peppers, celery sticks) for dipping

Preparation:
1. In a bowl, mix together the Greek yogurt, chopped cucumber, dill, lemon juice, and black pepper.
2. Chill in the refrigerator for at least 15 minutes before serving.
3. Serve with raw vegetables.
4. Prep Time: 10 minutes (+ 15 minutes chilling)

Nutritional Information (Per Serving):
- Calories: 60 kcal
- Potassium: 120 mg
- Phosphorus: 75 mg
- Sodium: 30 mg

- Protein: 5g
- Carbohydrates: 5g
- Fat: 2g
- Fiber: 1g

2. No-Salt-Added Popcorn

Ingredients:
1. 3 cups air-popped popcorn
2. 1 tbsp olive oil (optional for drizzling)
3. 1/2 tsp garlic powder (optional)
4. 1/2 tsp paprika (optional)
5. Ground black pepper (to taste)

Preparation:
1. Pop the popcorn kernels using an air popper or on the stove without added oil or salt.
2. If using, drizzle the popcorn with olive oil and sprinkle with garlic powder, paprika, and black pepper.
3. Toss the popcorn to evenly coat with seasonings.
4. Serve immediately.
5. Prep Time: 5 minutes

Nutritional Information (Per Serving):
- Calories: 80 kcal
- Potassium: 70 mg
- Phosphorus: 25 mg

- Sodium: 5 mg
- Protein: 2g
- Carbohydrates: 14g
- Fat: 4g
- Fiber: 3g

3. Apple Slices with Almond Butter

Ingredients:
1. 1 medium apple, sliced
2. 1 tbsp unsalted almond butter
3. Ground cinnamon (optional)

Preparation:
1. Slice the apple into wedges.
2. Spread almond butter onto each apple slice.
3. Sprinkle with ground cinnamon if desired.
4. Serve as a snack.
5. Prep Time: 5 minutes

Nutritional Information (Per Serving):
- Calories: 150 kcal
- Potassium: 200 mg
- Phosphorus: 35 mg
- Sodium: 2 mg
- Protein: 2g
- Carbohydrates: 20g
- Fat: 8g

- Fiber: 4g

4. Roasted Red Bell Pepper Hummus

Ingredients:
1. 1/2 cup canned chickpeas, drained and rinsed (low-sodium)
2. 1/4 cup roasted red bell peppers (unsalted, jarred or homemade)
3. 1 tbsp tahini (optional for flavor)
4. 1 clove garlic, minced
5. 1 tbsp lemon juice
6. 1 tbsp olive oil
7. Ground cumin and black pepper (to taste)
8. Fresh parsley for garnish (optional)
9. Sliced vegetables or low-sodium crackers for dipping

Preparation:
1. In a food processor, combine chickpeas, roasted red bell peppers, tahini, garlic, lemon juice, and olive oil.
2. Blend until smooth, adding a little water if needed to reach desired consistency.
3. Season with cumin and black pepper to taste.
4. Garnish with fresh parsley if desired.
5. Serve with sliced vegetables or low-sodium crackers.

6. Prep Time: 15 minutes

Nutritional Information (Per Serving):
- Calories: 120 kcal
- Potassium: 160 mg
- Phosphorus: 60 mg
- Sodium: 45 mg
- Protein: 3g
- Carbohydrates: 10g
- Fat: 8g
- Fiber: 3g

5. Zucchini Chips

Ingredients:
1. 1 medium zucchini, thinly sliced
2. 1 tbsp olive oil
3. 1 tsp dried oregano
4. Ground black pepper (to taste)

Preparation:
1. Preheat the oven to 225°F (110°C).
2. Place zucchini slices on a baking sheet lined with parchment paper.
3. Brush the slices with olive oil and sprinkle with dried oregano and black pepper.
4. Bake for 1.5 to 2 hours, turning halfway, until crispy.
5. Let cool slightly before serving.

6. Prep Time: 10 minutes (Active), 1.5 to 2 hours (Baking)

Nutritional Information (Per Serving):
- Calories: 90 kcal
- Potassium: 250 mg
- Phosphorus: 40 mg
- Sodium: 10 mg
- Protein: 1g
- Carbohydrates: 7g
- Fat: 7g
- Fiber: 1g

Beverages

1. Cucumber Mint Cooler

Ingredients:
1. 1/2 cup cucumber, peeled and sliced
2. 1 tbsp fresh mint leaves
3. 1 tsp lemon juice
4. 1 tsp honey (optional)
5. 1 cup cold water
6. Ice cubes

Preparation:
1. In a blender, combine cucumber slices, fresh mint, lemon juice, honey (if using), and cold water.
2. Blend until smooth.

3. Strain the mixture into a glass to remove any pulp.
4. Add ice cubes and garnish with a mint sprig if desired.
5. Serve chilled.
6. Prep Time: 5 minutes

Nutritional Information (Per Serving):
- Calories: 20 kcal
- Potassium: 50 mg
- Phosphorus: 5 mg
- Sodium: 2 mg
- Protein: 0g
- Carbohydrates: 5g
- Fat: 0g
- Fiber: 0g

2. Strawberry Lemon Infused Water

Ingredients:
1. 3-4 fresh strawberries, sliced
2. 1/2 lemon, thinly sliced
3. 4-5 fresh mint leaves (optional)
4. 1 liter water
5. Ice cubes

Preparation:
1. Place the strawberry slices, lemon slices, and mint leaves into a large pitcher.

2. Fill the pitcher with water and stir gently.
3. Refrigerate for at least 1 hour to allow the flavors to infuse.
4. Serve over ice.
5. Prep Time: 5 minutes (plus 1 hour for infusion)

Nutritional Information (Per Serving):
- Calories: 5 kcal
- Potassium: 10 mg
- Phosphorus: 1 mg
- Sodium: 1 mg
- Protein: 0g
- Carbohydrates: 1g
- Fat: 0g
- Fiber: 0g

3. Cranberry-Apple Spritzer

Ingredients:
1. 1/4 cup cranberry juice (100%, no added sugar)
2. 1/4 cup apple juice (100%, no added sugar)
3. 1/2 cup sparkling water (low sodium)
4. Ice cubes
5. Fresh cranberries or apple slices for garnish (optional)

Preparation:
1. In a glass, mix together cranberry juice and apple juice.
2. Add sparkling water and stir gently.
3. Add ice cubes and garnish with fresh cranberries or apple slices if desired.
4. Serve immediately.
5. Prep Time: 5 minutes

Nutritional Information (Per Serving):
- Calories: 60 kcal
- Potassium: 60 mg
- Phosphorus: 10 mg
- Sodium: 5 mg
- Protein: 0g
- Carbohydrates: 15g
- Fat: 0g
- Fiber: 0g

4. Herbal Iced Tea

Ingredients:
1. 1 herbal tea bag (such as chamomile, peppermint, or hibiscus)
2. 1 cup boiling water
3. 1 tsp honey (optional)
4. 1/2 cup cold water
5. Ice cubes
6. Lemon slice for garnish (optional)

Preparation:
1. Steep the herbal tea bag in boiling water for 5-7 minutes.
2. Remove the tea bag and let the tea cool slightly.
3. Add honey if desired, and stir until dissolved.
4. Mix in cold water and serve over ice.
5. Garnish with a lemon slice if desired.
6. Prep Time: 10 minutes

Nutritional Information (Per Serving):
- Calories: 20 kcal (with honey)
- Potassium: 5 mg
- Phosphorus: 0 mg
- Sodium: 0 mg
- Protein: 0g
- Carbohydrates: 5g
- Fat: 0g
- Fiber: 0g

5. Coconut Water Smoothie

Ingredients:
1. 1/2 cup unsweetened coconut water (check for low sodium options)
2. 1/4 cup fresh pineapple chunks
3. 1/4 cup fresh mango chunks
4. 1/4 cup ice cubes
5. 1 tsp fresh lime juice

Preparation:
1. In a blender, combine coconut water, pineapple chunks, mango chunks, ice cubes, and lime juice.
2. Blend until smooth.
3. Pour into a glass and serve immediately.
4. Prep Time: 5 minutes

Nutritional Information (Per Serving):
- Calories: 80 kcal
- Potassium: 100 mg
- Phosphorus: 15 mg
- Sodium: 20 mg
- Protein: 0g
- Carbohydrates: 20g
- Fat: 0g
- Fiber: 2g

1. Apple Cinnamon Oatmeal Cookies

Ingredients:
1. 1/2 cup unsalted butter, softened
2. 1/2 cup sugar
3. 1 egg
4. 1/2 tsp vanilla extract
5. 1 cup all-purpose flour
6. 1 cup rolled oats
7. 1/2 tsp baking powder
8. 1/2 tsp ground cinnamon
9. 1 small apple, peeled and finely chopped

Preparation:
1. Preheat the oven to 350°F (175°C) and line a baking sheet with parchment paper.
2. In a bowl, cream together the butter and sugar until light and fluffy.
3. Beat in the egg and vanilla extract.
4. In a separate bowl, mix together the flour, oats, baking powder, and cinnamon.
5. Gradually add the dry ingredients to the wet ingredients, mixing until just combined.
6. Fold in the chopped apple.

7. Drop spoonfuls of dough onto the prepared baking sheet.
8. Bake for 12-15 minutes, or until the edges are golden brown.
9. Cool on a wire rack before serving.
10. Prep Time: 20 minutes

Nutritional Information (Per Cookie):
- Calories: 100 kcal
- Potassium: 55 mg
- Phosphorus: 20 mg
- Sodium: 5 mg
- Protein: 1g
- Carbohydrates: 14g
- Fat: 4g
- Fiber: 1g

2. Vanilla Rice Pudding

Ingredients:
1. 1/2 cup white rice (cooked)
2. 1 cup rice milk (unsweetened, low-sodium)
3. 1/4 cup sugar
4. 1/2 tsp vanilla extract
5. 1/4 tsp ground cinnamon (optional)

Preparation:
1. In a saucepan, combine cooked rice, rice milk, and sugar.

2. Cook over medium heat, stirring frequently, until the mixture thickens (about 10-15 minutes).
3. Remove from heat and stir in vanilla extract.
4. Sprinkle with ground cinnamon if desired.
5. Serve warm or chilled.
6. Prep Time: 20 minutes

Nutritional Information (Per Serving):
- Calories: 130 kcal
- Potassium: 30 mg
- Phosphorus: 20 mg
- Sodium: 25 mg
- Protein: 2g
- Carbohydrates: 27g
- Fat: 1g
- Fiber: 0g

3. Blueberry Sorbet

Ingredients:
1. 2 cups fresh or frozen blueberries (low potassium)
2. 1/4 cup sugar
3. 1/4 cup water
4. 1 tbsp lemon juice

Preparation:
1. In a saucepan, combine sugar and water, and heat until the sugar is fully dissolved.
2. In a blender, puree the blueberries with the lemon juice.
3. Mix the blueberry puree with the sugar syrup.
4. Pour the mixture into a shallow dish and freeze for 2-3 hours, stirring every 30 minutes to break up ice crystals.
5. Serve once fully frozen.
6. Prep Time: 10 minutes (active), 2-3 hours (freezing)

Nutritional Information (Per Serving):
- Calories: 80 kcal
- Potassium: 50 mg
- Phosphorus: 10 mg
- Sodium: 0 mg
- Protein: 0g
- Carbohydrates: 20g
- Fat: 0g
- Fiber: 2g

4. Coconut Macaroons

Ingredients:
1. 1   1/2   cups   unsweetened   shredded coconut
2. 1/4 cup sugar
3. 2 egg whites
4. 1/2 tsp vanilla extract

Preparation:
1. Preheat the oven to 325°F (165°C) and line a baking sheet with parchment paper.
2. In a bowl, mix together the shredded coconut and sugar.
3. In a separate bowl, beat the egg whites until stiff peaks form.
4. Fold the egg whites into the coconut mixture, then add vanilla extract.
5. Drop spoonfuls of the mixture onto the prepared baking sheet.
6. Bake for 15-20 minutes, or until golden brown.
7. Cool on a wire rack before serving.
8. Prep Time: 20 minutes

Nutritional Information (Per Macaroon):
- Calories: 80 kcal
- Potassium: 50 mg
- Phosphorus: 15 mg

- Sodium: 20 mg
- Protein: 1g
- Carbohydrates: 8g
- Fat: 5g
- Fiber: 2g

5. Peach and Berry Parfait

Ingredients:
1. 1/2 cup peaches, diced (fresh or canned in water)
2. 1/4 cup mixed berries (such as blueberries and raspberries)
3. 1/2 cup plain Greek yogurt (unsweetened, low-sodium)
4. 1 tsp honey (optional)

Preparation:
1. In a glass or bowl, layer the diced peaches and mixed berries.
2. Top with Greek yogurt.
3. Drizzle with honey if desired.
4. Serve immediately.
5. Prep Time: 5 minutes

Nutritional Information (Per Serving):
- Calories: 100 kcal
- Potassium: 150 mg
- Phosphorus: 70 mg
- Sodium: 30 mg

- Protein: 5g
- Carbohydrates: 15g
- Fat: 2g
- Fiber: 3g

14-Day Exercise Plan

This plan focuses on low-impact exercises that can be performed safely while providing benefits such as improved circulation, muscle strength, and overall well-being.

General Guidelines:
1. Consultation: Always consult with a healthcare provider before starting any exercise program.
2. Intensity: Keep the exercises low-impact and moderate in intensity. Listen to the body and avoid overexertion.
3. Hydration: Stay hydrated, but follow fluid intake guidelines as prescribed by the doctor.
4. Warm-Up and Cool-Down: Begin each session with a 5-10 minute warm-up (light walking or stretching) and end with a 5-10 minute cool-down.

Day 1: Gentle Stretching and Walking
Warm-Up: 5 minutes of light walking
Exercise:
- 10 minutes of gentle stretching (neck rolls, shoulder shrugs, arm circles, leg stretches)
- 15 minutes of slow to moderate walking

Cool-Down: 5 minutes of slow walking and deep breathing

Day 2: Seated Exercises
Warm-Up: 5 minutes of arm and leg movements while seated
Exercise:
- 10 minutes of seated leg lifts (10 reps per leg)
- 10 minutes of seated arm exercises (arm circles, bicep curls with light weights or water bottles)

Cool-Down: 5 minutes of seated stretches (reach forward, side stretches)

Day 3: Rest or Light Activity
- Light Activity: Engage in light household activities like gardening, tidying up, or a short walk.

Day 4: Low-Impact Aerobics
Warm-Up: 5 minutes of light marching in place

Exercise:
- 20 minutes of low-impact aerobics (marching in place, side steps, gentle arm movements)

Cool-Down: 5 minutes of stretching and deep breathing

Day 5: Balance and Flexibility
Warm-Up: 5 minutes of light walking
Exercise:
- 10 minutes of balance exercises (standing on one leg, heel-to-toe walking)
- 10 minutes of flexibility exercises (gentle stretches for legs, back, and shoulders)

Cool-Down: 5 minutes of seated stretching

Day 6: Seated Yoga
Warm-Up: 5 minutes of deep breathing and seated arm stretches
Exercise:
- 20 minutes of seated yoga (gentle twists, seated forward bends, neck stretches)

Cool-Down: 5 minutes of seated meditation or relaxation

Day 7: Rest or Light Activity
- Light Activity: Engage in light activities like walking, gardening, or gentle stretching.

Day 8: Strength Training
Warm-Up: 5 minutes of light walking or marching in place
Exercise:
- 10 minutes of upper body strength exercises (use light weights or resistance bands)
- 10 minutes of lower body strength exercises (leg lifts, seated squats)
Cool-Down: 5 minutes of stretching

Day 9: Walking and Flexibility
Warm-Up: 5 minutes of slow walking
Exercise:
- 15-20 minutes of walking at a comfortable pace
- 10 minutes of flexibility exercises (gentle stretches)
Cool-Down: 5 minutes of slow walking and deep breathing

Day 10: Rest or Light Activity
- Light Activity: Engage in light activities such as walking or simple household chores.

Day 11: Seated Exercises
Warm-Up: 5 minutes of gentle seated stretches
Exercise:
- 20 minutes of seated exercises (arm raises, leg lifts, seated marches)

Cool-Down: 5 minutes of deep breathing and seated stretches

Day 12: Balance and Core Stability
Warm-Up: 5 minutes of light walking
Exercise:
- 10 minutes of balance exercises (heel-to-toe walking, standing on one leg)
- 10 minutes of core exercises (seated leg lifts, seated core twists)

Cool-Down: 5 minutes of stretching

Day 13: Low-Impact Aerobics
Warm-Up: 5 minutes of light marching in place
Exercise:
- 20 minutes of low-impact aerobics (side steps, gentle arm movements, marching in place)

Cool-Down: 5 minutes of stretching and deep breathing

Day 14: Rest or Light Activity
- Light Activity: Engage in a light walk, gentle stretching, or a relaxing activity like meditation.

Tips for Success

1. Listen to Your Body: If you feel fatigued or experience any discomfort, stop the exercise and rest.
2. Stay Consistent: Aim to incorporate physical activity into your daily routine, even if it's just a short walk.
3. Modify as Needed: Adjust the intensity, duration, and type of exercise based on your comfort level and doctor's recommendations.

CONCLUSION

Managing stage 4 chronic kidney disease (CKD) is a complex journey that requires a thoughtful approach to nutrition and lifestyle. This book has been designed as a comprehensive guide to help seniors navigate the dietary challenges associated with this advanced stage of CKD. Through detailed food lists, carefully crafted recipes, and evidence-based recommendations, our goal is to empower you with the knowledge and tools needed to support your kidney health.

This book has provided you with a wide variety of kidney-friendly foods, categorized by their nutrient content, making it easier to plan meals that meet your dietary needs. From low-sodium vegetables and fruits to low-phosphorus grains and proteins, the food lists offer options that are both nutritious and suitable for your condition.

The meal planning tips provided are intended to help you organize your grocery shopping, prepare meals in advance, and maintain a balanced diet that supports your health. These tips, along with the nutritional information provided for each recipe, give you the tools to track your nutrient intake and make informed decisions about your diet.

Staying Informed and Adaptive
Living with stage 4 CKD requires ongoing attention to your health and diet. The information in this book is a starting point for managing your condition, but it's essential to stay informed and adaptable. Regular consultations with your healthcare team, including your nephrologist and dietitian, are crucial to ensure that your diet continues to meet your evolving health needs.

This book encourages you to be proactive in your health management. By understanding the reasons behind dietary recommendations and staying committed to a kidney-friendly diet, you can take control of your health and work towards better outcomes.

At its core, this book is about supporting your quality of life. A well-managed diet can make a significant difference in how you feel on a day-to-day basis, helping to reduce symptoms, manage complications, and maintain your strength and energy levels.

We hope that this book has provided you with valuable insights and practical resources to make the journey with stage 4 CKD more manageable. Remember that each individual's experience with CKD is unique, and your diet should be personalized to your specific needs and preferences.

The road with stage 4 CKD may be challenging, but with the right tools and mindset, you can navigate it effectively. Use this book as an ongoing resource, referring back to the food lists, recipes, and guidelines as needed. Stay engaged with your healthcare team, be mindful of your dietary choices, and most importantly, listen to your body.

Your commitment to a kidney-friendly diet is a crucial step towards managing your health and improving your quality of life. I hope that the knowledge and guidance provided in this book will help you make positive, lasting changes that support your well-being.

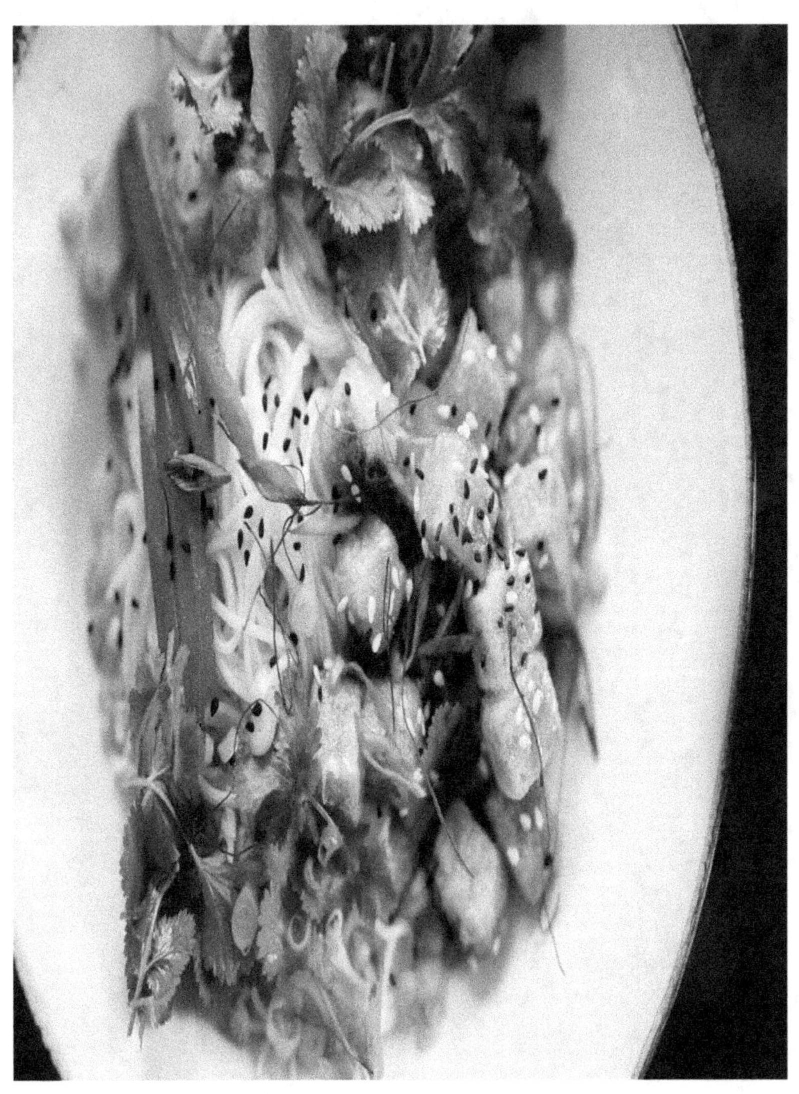

241 KIDNEY DISEASE DIET FOOD LIST FOR SENIORS ON STAGE 4